# TIME MACHINE

## A program for restoring body, mind and spirit for the over fifties'

## Elizabeth Kaziro

## Infinity Spirituality

www.infinityspirituality.com.au

**ISBN** 1492794104

**It's never too late to become what you might have been –**

**George Eliot**

# ACKNOWLEDGEMENTS

My sincere thanks to the four contributors who generously provided biographies of their own experiences of discovering exercise in mature life and then encouraging others to find the exercise pathway as exciting and rewarding as they have – Diane Gosden, David Gosden, John 'Sparrow' Dowse and Ann Cusack.

And deep appreciation for those who have proof-read the publication and given advice and support.

# CONTENTS

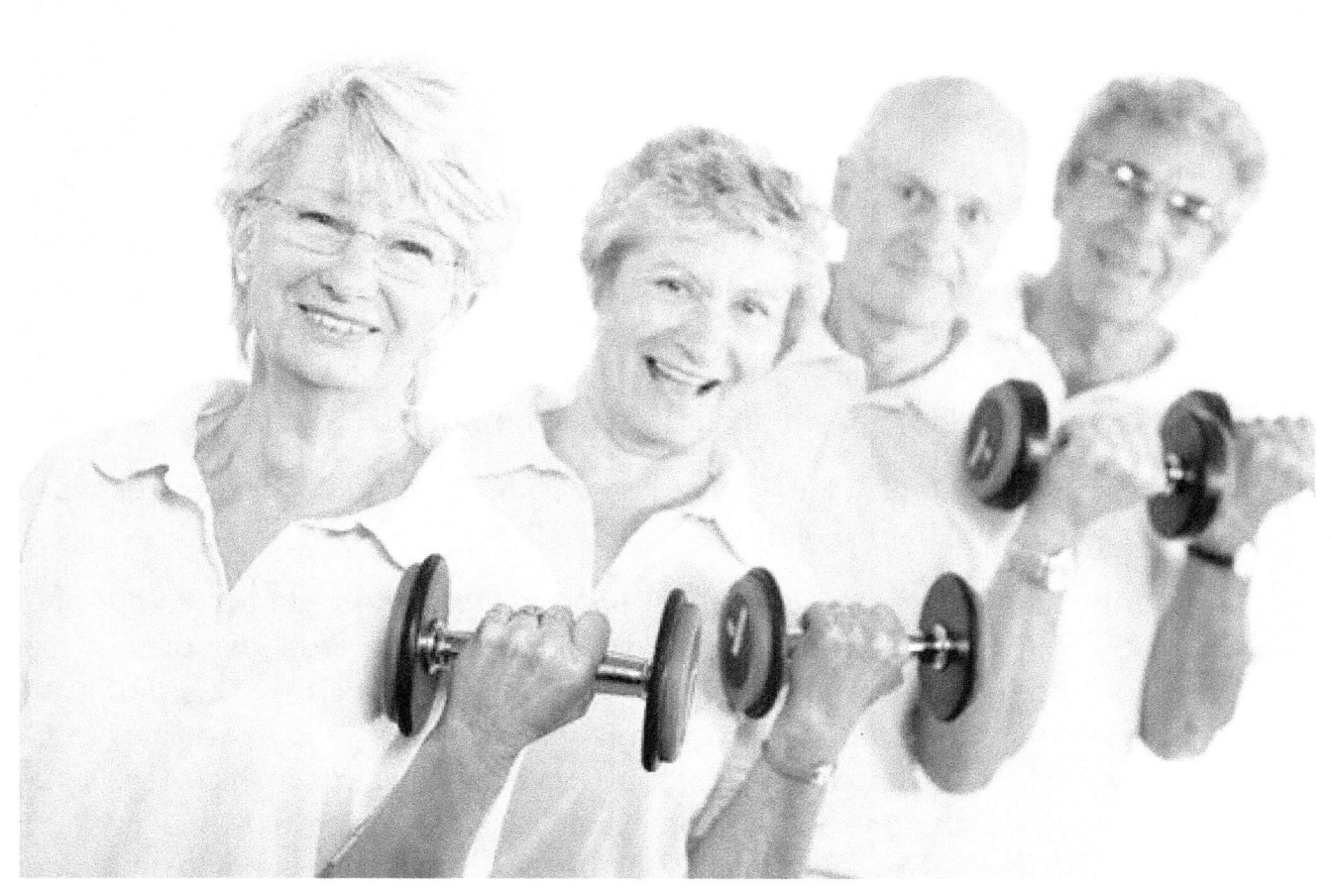

# TIME MACHINE

## PART ONE:   Achieving Fitness After 50

### Introduction:  Over Fifty Client?

The breakdown of hormonal production brings about changes in energy, bone density and with a sedentary lifestyle, muscle strength, flexibility, range of joint movement and cardiorespiratory fitness diminishes. However, age is an excuse, not a reason to slip further into immobility. Even the style of 'gentle exercise' understates the capacity of the body to reinstitute health and activity.  Unless a client has a definite medical condition, strength and endurance can be worked up to and equal to that

of a young adult.  And if there is a defined medical condition, prescribed exercise will help to alleviate the condition.

Although the osteoclasts which break down bone cells accelerate after thirty five years of age, the building blocks of the cells, osteoblasts can be stimulated to reform bone by high impact exercise.  This is not the gentle swinging of a limb while grasping a chair.  It is more likely to be weights, high impact aerobics or kickboxing where multiple skills are needed such as speed and precision in hand and leg movements and a great deal of concentration. But beware of further wearing out older joints!

Postural analysis after fifty is also a great bonus for adjusting long standing problems especially if a client has been crouched over a computer for years.  What are the give-aways for looking aged?  Posture would definitely be in the fore with lack of muscle tone, expanding midriff and neglect of other really important areas.  A person doesn't need plastic surgery – just skin care, hair care, teeth maintenance and a commitment to grooming that a twenty year old has.  For the rest – it is right and good to age gracefully – knowing that the best has been done!

This is a program about finding body, soul and spirit again and making the years over fifty challenging, healthy and rich in relationships.

**Age-related Health Problems:**

Inactivity and weight gain are associated with conditions of age such as osteoporosis, impotence, insomnia and diabetes. The foundation of health in older age is the overcoming of inflexibility through stretching and a minimum of 30 minutes of physical activity daily. Moderate exercise will also reduce blood pressure, positively alter the blood lipid profile and reduce insensitivity to glucose – acting as a prevention to mature-onset diabetes.

By limiting fats and adhering to a healthy diet, it is considered that 30-50% of cancers can be prevented. As well as plenty of fibre, water – oily fish such as mackerel, salmon, sardines and tuna protect against heart disease by escalating high-density lipoproteins which are extremely valuable. Heart disease or strokes can be flagged by the danger of high blood pressure.

Osteoporosis can be detected through bone density scans and is also associated with fractures when falls occur with the over 70's. Fish oils are important as they help lower blood cholesterol levels, ease arthritis and improve circulation. There has also been research to link Vitamin E intake with reduced risk of heart disease and prostate cancer.

A trainer can monitor body composition and essentially body fat either in the gym or it can be carried out by the client at home with body monitoring devices. Even if weight is maintained in older age at the same level as in the 30's, muscle may have declined while the percentage of body fat has increased. This creates a greater risk of certain cancers, diabetes and heart disease.

The suppression of the thirst-mechanism after 50 years of age can result in serious dehydration and is also linked to bowel and prostate cancer, kidney stones and gall stones. 6-8 glasses of water per day is recommended to remedy this situation.

Mammograms for women and bowel cancer tests for men and women every 2 years assist in the early detection of cancers and help to save many lives. Stroke victims are also assisted by practising T'ai Chi to stimulate body awareness and brain-eye co-ordination.

While osteoporosis is improved by a reasonable degree of impact in exercise, the risk of arthritis is greater in the older age group and the trainer might favour a low impact activity such as swimming or walking. Also T'ai Chi does not stress the legs and ankles.

Exercising the mind is also essential which can be by reading, cross-words or major projects which require responsibility and planning.

## Developing Fitness & Rehab Programs for Seniors

With an increased ageing population in most of the Western world, prospective health care costs for over 50 year olds take up a significant proportion of the health care budget. There are no real expectations that our sedentary ageing population will in any way change their ways without significant encouragement and incentives from different levels of government and for medical reasons. The opportunity to explore fitness options through an array of facilities and with trained supervision is not taken up by the majority of the mature population for a variety of reasons. These include cost of equipment, trainers; low confidence and self esteem; lack of knowledge of the benefits of fitness programs; absence of local facilities and the need for continuing support and advice in creating healthy lifestyles.

Nevertheless, it can be established that a focussed recruitment of the mature population in a local setting will generate higher health and fitness levels – by this means increasing mobility, mental and physical standards and reducing overall needs for high cost medical care and medication in the long run. Increased longevity of the population will require the establishment of local fitness facilities which will be as important as the local library and child health care centre. Some programs do exist in centres for 'Seniors' and hospitals but the intensity of the programs and their purpose will vary and also the availability of places can be scarce. What is needed is an outreach into the community to establish fitness and health needs, the setting up of a pilot program to provide substantive material for further private organisational and government policy decision-making on fitness programs for the targeted age groups. Such fitness centres could also provide practical data for research.

In Australia, present government legislation regarding health claim benefits for gym membership was cut out at the end of 2003. Provider numbers (and health benefit claims) cover such health programs as stress management, diabetes education, childbirth education, quit smoking, asthma education, weight loss programs, accidentrevention/safety (first aid and swimming classes). However, no fitness programs covering cardiorespiratory and resistance, flexibility and balance training are covered for the general population. In spite of increased research into the benefits of exercise in relation to the effects of ageing, rehabilitation and depression - political decision-making has been to the contrary. Some facilities such as the Area Health & Leisure Centre at Royal Prince Alfred Hospital, Sydney were also scaled down. This facility trained a number of referred rehabilitation patients from the hospital and older people who had graduated from the 'Strong Program' at Balmain Hospital.

There are many established programs which also generate research such as the through Health Sciences, at the University of Sydney, the Lifestyle Centre at the University of New South Wales and at Tufts University, Boston. The Victorian Council for the Ageing also has sought to expand existing facilities with exercise programs for mature populations. It is anticipated that medical practitioners will be receptive to prescribing fitness programs if they are sufficiently conversant with the benefits and nature of exercise prescription. Accreditation and/or qualifications of fitness trainers and exercise physicians will contribute to confident referrals by medical practitioners.

Identification, education and training in fitness and health issues for the mature population over 50 years of age will significantly impact upon mobility, lifestyle and health care costs. Community outreach and education can reinforce the need for individual commitment to regular programs. In an age of specialisation, it is hoped that this publication will reach the people most affected by the ageing process as well as their carers, medical advisers and allied health professionals. Trainers and exercise physicians have an excellent opportunity to turn around the lives of people over 50 and to motivate them to maintain mobility, balance as well as to prevent and heal metabolic disorders, cardio-respiratory ailments and to help alleviate depression.

**DEFINITION OF TERMS:**

**Cardiovascular Exercise:**

Movement which involves the use of the large muscle groups. Oxygen is used as a source of energy to create movement – strengthening the heart, lungs and circulatory system.

**Resistance Training:**

Resistance training involves exerting a force to enable movement or application of tension to a weight, resulting in enhanced muscular strength and endurance. The intensity and repetition of the applied force, determines whether muscular strength or endurance are being built up.

**Flexibility Programs:**

A program designed to optimize mobility and enhance elasticity of muscles, while maintaining stability of the joints. Flexibility diminishes with age and with a loss of elasticity in the connective tissue surrounding the muscles. Combined with inactive lifestyle – mobility becomes limited.

## Consultative Professional Networks

Fitness trainers need to be able to identify physiological or psychological limitations to exercise via PAR-Q (Physical Activity Readiness Questionnaire), physical assessment and psychological screening. Appropriate allied health professionals and medical advisers may be networked and their roles identified in assessing the fitness or health status of older adult clients and in conducting exercise programs. For example:

- Exercise scientists assess and prescribe rehabilitation programs;

- Dieticians assist with nutritional counselling;

- Counsellors provide motivational and emotional support;

- Psychologists assess and treat mental health problems;

- Osteopaths, physiotherapists and masseurs promote rehabilitation through musculoskeletal therapy;

- Medical practitioners assess general health conditions, make diagnosis and prognosis and may refer on to medical specialists for specific disorders.

A fitness trainer may identify an older client with diminished balance skills and would then refer the client to their medical practitioner. Before prescribing exercise, the fitness trainer would request exercise advice from the medical practitioner with the client's written consent.

In determining the risk status of an older adult client before prescribing exercise, the fitness trainer should ask the client to fill in the PAR-Q. An older client can be excluded from participation in exercise if the client does not complete or sign-off on the PAR-Q or does not give written informed consent. It is also inadvisable for an older client to be prescribed exercise if he/she answers 'yes' to one or more of items on the PAR-Q.

Before the assessment it is advisable to ask the client to wear appropriate loose clothing and to have no intake of food or caffeine 2-3 hours before the assessment.

If an older client needs to be referred after they have been excluded from participation in an exercise program, it is essential to explain the legal obligations i.e. duty of care and any ethical concerns, using empathy in the situation.

## CHAPTER ONE:  Tests for Fitness

### Look Good – Feel Good?

Depending upon hormonal changes – sometimes people genuinely don't care how they look as they get older.  But of course, other people do care, especially those closest to the client.  If the client believed that a youthful and healthy body was an option then most likely it would be something worth working for.  If we look around we can find some very inspiring examples of people well over fifty who have continued to swim, run and workout in the gym regularly.  Or perhaps they have taken it up after fifty.   There are several mature fitness pioneers featured, who continue to see fitness as a lifestyle goal and serve as a great motivation to others.

There is no substitute for experiencing well-being – that feeling of peace, fitness and confidence which allows for anything to be taken on.  Physical fitness combines with the ability to avoid common diseases of age, such as heart disease, hypertension, diabetes II, lipidaemia, obesity, depression and osteoporosis.  If these diseases are present and at an early stage, the effect of exercising can actually reduce and sometimes eliminate the condition.

What is needed for the client initially, is a knowledge of exercise programs, nutritional input and a firm commitment to taking responsibility for the body and all its workings.

### Tests for Fitness

Pre-test screening is undertaken by many gymnasiums for the over-fifty population who are embarking on the adventure of fitness training.  Fitness testing is regarded as essential in all ages but especially in the senior age bracket.  The Swedish exercise physiologist, Olaf Astrand regarded inactivity as a far greater danger than actual physical exercise.  Setting a gauge for endurance goals and measuring any improvements will form the basis of planning an exercise program.  Motivational tools are often related to age, blood pressure and medical history, obesity and may be mental health problems including depression. Clearance from a general practitioner might also be needed.

Safe exercise prescription can be undertaken by a skilled exercise physiologist or trainer who may also use a safety questionnaire to reveal the client's self-perception of his/her own health, weight, general fitness and how the client wants to go forward with planning a new fitness model. Some of the areas which are checked on the list would be high cholesterol, prescribed medications, arthritis, hernia, asthma, diabetes, dizziness, epilepsy, back or joint conditions, chest pain and past and present injuries to the body. Above all, what does the client expect to gain from a fitness program?

### Techniques of Fitness Assessment:

Some common tests are for cardiorespiratory endurance, muscular strength and endurance, muscular endurance on its own and flexibility.

### Cardiorespiratory endurance (VO2max):

VO2max looks at oxygen distribution throughout the body and measures its capacity to be transported to and used by functioning muscles. Poor fitness would be exhibited in a middle-aged man through VO2max at say 26 ml/kg/min. On the other hand an elite athlete might reach 92 ml/kg/min during an endurance training session. Gyms and clinics usually run the test by means of a bicycle ergometer, bench stepping or a treadmill. Others might gauge VO2 max after a short run.

### Muscular Strength & Endurance:

One of the hardest tests for older people is sit-ups which measure abdominal strength and even harder to avoid is the use of the hip flexors. Arms can be folded across the chest or on the floor, or some even prefer to hold the feet while a dynamometer measures handgrip strength, back lift and leg lift strength. Tensiometers are also used to indicate strength within a number of muscle groups. Weight lifting allows for the measurement of power and strength in relative and absolute terms.

## Muscular Strength & Endurance:

The measure of arm, shoulder and back strength endurance is best done by chin-ups and these are especially difficult for women. Flexed arm hangs measure forearm, biceps and upper back muscle endurance. Pushups are a useful measure for chest, shoulder and triceps muscular endurance while once again sit-ups measure abdominal endurance.

## Muscular Endurance:

Another difficult test for the over fifties is the 'sit and reach test' which measures static flexibility at the hip joint. Leighton's flexometer also has a wider scope of measuring the flexibility of all joints in degrees.

## Measuring Body Fatness:

MRI or Magnetic Resonance Imagery and CAT scan, Computerised Anthropometric Tomography are used regularly to determine body fatness. The main anthropometric measures are height, weight, girth and body composition. However, to get back to the gym or the clinic, special skinfold callipers are the usual method of assessing skinfold measurements. Height-to-weight ratios are also often used as a combined measure of obesity or overweight. The biceps, triceps, subscapular (on the back), suprailia (above the hip bone), mid-anterior thigh, abdomen and chest provide adequate sites for the skin fold testing. The sum of averaged skin folds are converted to percent body fat using tables. Although not desirable nor healthy, older men and women have approximately 5-10% more fat than younger people.

Once exercise is taken up, the transformation and evaluation of alterations to body shape might be seen through girth measurements. It is important to remember that there will be differences in measurement of WHR (Waist-to-hip ratio) in men and women considering android and gynoid factors. WHR is calculated by dividing an individual's girth at the waist by their hip girth. Women who measure over 0.8 and men over 0.9 need to understand that they are at a greater health risk.

Simple girth measurements can evaluate changes in body shape and provide you with excellent feedback from the results of exercising and reduced fat intakes. Chest, waist, hips, thigh, calf and upper arm measurements can also document changes due to transformation of lifestyle.

**Blood Pressure:**

Anyone who records a blood pressure measure of 140/90 has borderline hypertension (high blood pressure) and should consult a physician for further medical advice, especially if the person is intending to take up exercise (National Heart Foundation). The contraction phase (systolic) and the relaxation phase (diastolic) form the two measures of blood pressure with the acceptable range being 120 +-19 and 80 +-10. Blood pressure can be measured by the auscultatory method, using a stethoscope.

Fitness is also be tested in the most simple ways such as a 'talk-test' – a monitoring process undertaken through communication during exercise

Depression can also be a sign of lack of fitness. Challenge often diminishes depression, and while people over fifty are more conservative when it comes to new lifestyles and exertion, they deserve to be given exciting new opportunities.

## CHAPTER TWO:  Exercises for Daily Balance & Ageing

Of special concern in the ageing process is the need to prevent imbalance and the risk of injury through falling as well as maintaining mobility.  Optimal balance is achieved through the systems of the body such as visual, vestibular and proprioception.

The ocular nerve receives, via the retina filtration of images, information which is important to the visual or reticular systems.  The eyes achieve triangulation to gauge depth perception and thus determine any potential risks or obstacles and compromised sight can affect the function of this system.

When glasses are removed or where a person has a sight disorder, some postural changes can be exacerbated, for example with asymmetrical weight shift left or right and with forward head posture. To also measure the visual input for alignment and balance, assessment can be done with eyes open and eyes closed if there is no sight impairment.  If  an elderly person cannot visually line the body up with a static external reference point – there must be some expectation that posture will be adversely effected.

### Vestibular:

The rate and extent of head movement, forward and backwards is determined by the vestibulocochlear nerve which also carries information for balance.  The head relates to gravity with a three dimensional orientation and information is provided to the brain by vestibular middle ear section.  It is made up of three fluid filled semi-circular canals.

Middle ear infections from flu can also affect a person's balance and delay messages of balance information reaching the brain.  Any change in the integrity of the vestibular system can alter balance.

### Proprioception:

Peripheral receptors acquire stimuli which are converted to a neural signal which is transmitted along the afferent pathway to the Central Nervous System and accordingly forms proprioception.

When information is required to sustain muscle tone and perform complex co-ordinated exercises, proprioceptive receptors give essential information to the Central Nervous System

## Dynamic & Static Stability Relating to Overcoming Ageing Effects:

### Static:

Firstly, to establish a mode of stability without taking into account complex movements, trainers usually devise static postures which can be undertaken in short periods of time and utilise specific muscle functions. Base floor exercises can be also used as well as implementing a fitball to increase variety and intensity of exercises.

### Dynamic:

Progression can then be made from the static to dynamic states which improve the functional stability of an older person and as the body ages creates surety and confidence. For the frail elderly one of the greatest risks to health and wellbeing, is the danger of falls and the loss of confidence and mobility once that has occurred.

There is a lot more to walking than imagined, with multiple joints through every angle of movement employed. Exercises require efficiency, the use of specific muscles, the retention of joint alignment and the acceptable conscription of muscles.

## POSTURE:

As mentioned earlier, posture is one of the first give-aways of ageing. It can be influenced by many factors which might include injuries, personality, emotions, genetic factors, weight and life-long sedentary occupations. It is what the body tells us about personal attitude and position and should be an efficient yet minimal tool.

### Posture is a Body Language Cue:

Posture expresses the personality, inner health and emotional life. Depression often causes a person to minimalize breathing and as the respiratory system becomes shallow so does the interaction with the endocrine and immune systems. Shoulders may round and the chest sags while others adopt a forward head position. Sliding down on the chair so that the lower back engages almost with the seat instead of the buttocks is a common postural fault.

On the other hand accidents may result in the shortening or imbalance of a leg length and genetic imbalances of even 1 cm can cause postural problems. Shortening of the hamstrings and ligamentous tension and muscle tightness will affect the hips and back. When the knees are affected walking also becomes difficult. Chronic pain can ensue from these imbalances and if the postural imbalance is not corrected it is often re-enforced.

**The Ideal Posture:**

To assess and correct posture – observation is carried out with the musculoskeletal systems starting with the supine, side and prone lying positions followed by the standing position to find distortions with posture and core of the body.

- There should be minimal work by the muscles and alignment to achieve balance, symmetry and poise.

- The position of the plumb line should be through middle of the ear, shoulders, femur and slight anterior to the lateral malleolus.

**Standing:**

Biomechanical efficiency creates the criteria for assessing correct anatomical postures. *Feldenkreis* has described this as the position from where all movement, in any direction, starts and finishes with the least possible effort.

*Humans, existing as the only erect species in the presence of gravity, are designed to have our primary weight-bearing joints vertically aligned and horizontally parallel with each other and with the ground. Thus, shoulders, hips, knees and ankles line up over and above one another from the side, while the front and rear, shoulders are level, hips level, knees point straight ahead, and feet are straight ahead and held at the width of the hips sockets. The right and left sides, being mirror images of one another in both form and function, each bear half the weight. This creates a perfect four-socket-position frame with a right angle at each primary weight-bearing joint. This right-angled design confers the greatest structural integrity (neutrality) to the human form in relation to the force of gravity. (Geoff Gluckman, Muscle Balance and Function Development (as Printed in B.C. Massage Practitioner, Fall, 1995))*

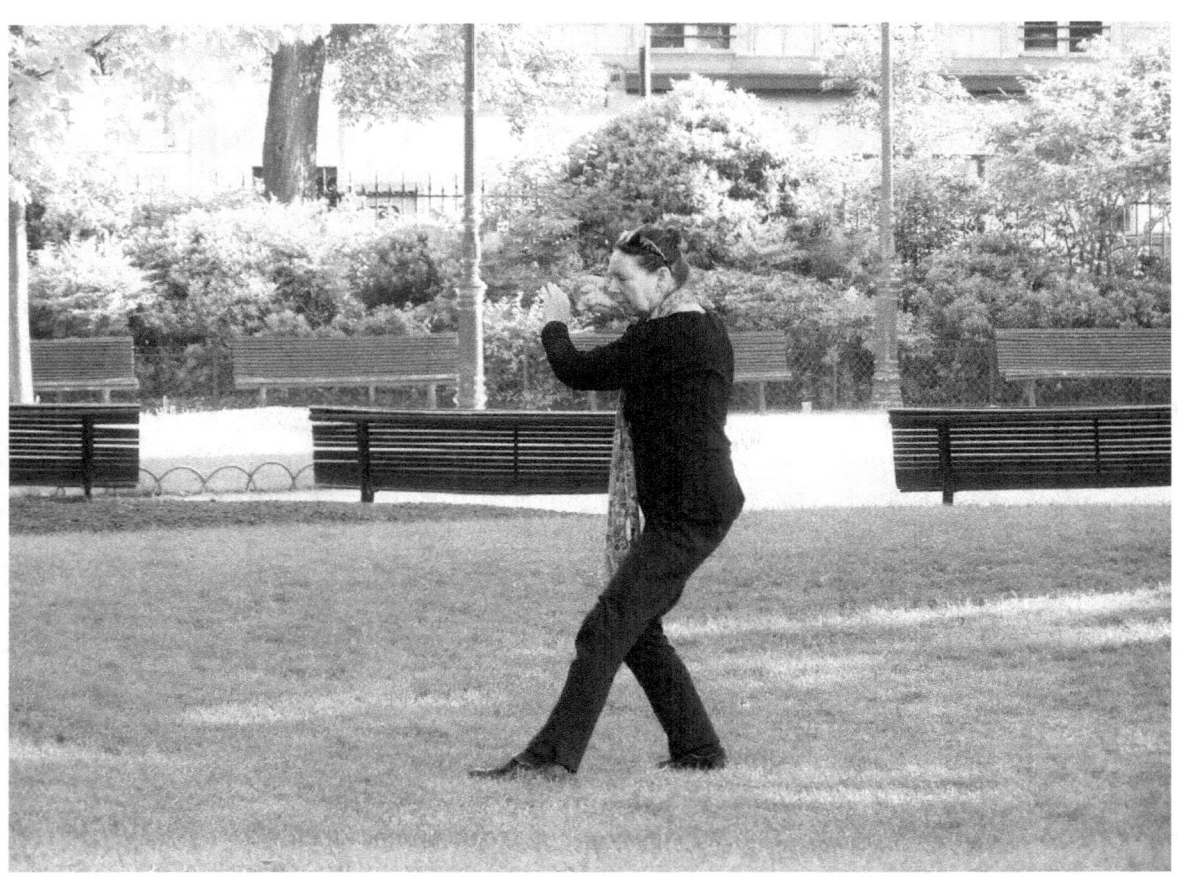

I began to learn and practice Tai Chi in earnest about 10 years ago, when I was in my late fifties.

It has many benefits for health. It improves balance, flexibility and muscle strength, especially in the legs. It also has mental and emotional benefits through the relaxation and concentration that accompany the movements. As many people have said of Tai Chi - it is a moving meditation.

Tai Chi originated in China. Originally, all of the movements were martial arts movements, which of course required good balance and coordination. Later, it was realised that when performed slowly and in a relaxed manner, there were many health benefits that could be gained from practising the movements and positions. It was from this realisation that the form of Tai Chi with which most people are familiar, emerged. This is Tai Chi Slow Form - the slow and graceful steps and patterns of movements that can be seen in any public space in China and Hong Kong, and increasingly also in Australia.

There are many schools of Tai Chi, but all will emphasise the relationship of the opposite but complementary and alternating nature of yin and yang in the movements. In doing Tai Chi, one becomes much more aware of where one's weight is centred, eg. is there more weight in one foot than in the other? Is the distribution of weight in the legs more in the toe or the heel, or in the middle of the feet? All of this, as well as the positions themselves, improve awareness of balance. In addition, with enhanced relaxation in the body, the energy of a movement can travel effortlessly through the body, improving circulation.

I find that at 68 years of age, the practise of Tai Chi has become an integral and indispensable part of my life. I include a photograph of myself on holiday in Paris to prove it. Even there, I found a great place to do some practice.

Diane Gosden.

## CHAPTER THREE:  Strength & Resistance Training

The preliminaries have been settled!  Fitness levels have been established, the client  has been cleared medically and limitations understood.  The personal trainer or gymnasium instructor designs a program  -  goals can be set and supervision and monitoring of a program can commence.  Once experience is gained, the client might want to be more independent while others feel that a trainer gives them additional motivation to achieve the goals and to confirm changes.

Fitness targets are set on current fitness levels and also whether the client  wants to achieve a lean body weight, become a body builder or help to correct a medical condition.   A fitness instructor will write up a program that could cover different fitness outcomes and would take into account any injuries or illnesses.  The need to supervise and monitor the rate of fitness adaptations will take into account a natural plateau that is reached after about four weeks, so that further planning will produce the desired changes and reach the fitness goal.  Motivation is very important to keep a program going and so although it might come from a trainer or the transformation taking place, individuals also need to look at the whole spectrum of fitness and ageing to understand the benefits gained.

**Resistance Training for Seniors**

Normal daily activities are sometimes the greatest challenges for seniors and any program designed for them should seek to emphasise an improvement in quality of life for the individual.  This would mean producing more energy, strength and stamina to help maintain independence – build up muscle tissue and a sense of well-being.

Muscle strength even for those elite athletes does not last beyond 60 to 65.  Fatigue brings on immobility and immobility gives way to falls and fractures.  Even rising from a chair can be a significant challenge, with a strong person taking 0.6 seconds while a weak person may take 6 seconds.   By developing strength in the lower extremities, calf muscles, ankles, quads and hips, much can be done to avoid obstacles in fall injuries.  It is surprising that 40% of people over 65, experience at least one fall a year and particularly in the frail elderly – falls may be a cause of death.

The chest, trunk and back muscles should be included in any exercise program even though there may be emphasis on mobility and the lower extremities. The knee and hip extensors have many functional purposes while the dorsiflexors of the foot assist with walking and leg strength can diminish quickly – so all these groups must be well maintained. Elderly people also use their arms more even if they are immobile, consequently strengthening them and building muscle.

One of the most important things is the regulation of rhythmic breathing – making sure exhalation during the exertion phase of a lift is emphasised to avoid breath holding. This can increase blood pressure while pulse may decrease. As many older people have high blood pressure and heart disorders, this is a much safer protocol to avoid cardiovascular functional disorders.

In working out a resistance program for the over fifties, there are greater benefits of training this age group to work at 60-80% maximum capacity. Injury is avoided by working slowly from a low weight to heavier weights. If a maximum capacity of 80% is reached then that should be sufficient. Within the muscle group selected, 6-10 exercises can be selected. 1-2 sets should be enough with 8-12 repetitions.

**Suggested exercises:**

- Toe Tapping

- Bench Press

- Seated Military Press Leg Extension

- Leg Extension

- Cable Hip Extension

- Leg Curl

- Abdominal Crunch

- Bicep Curl

- Controlled Back Extension Lat Pull Down

    (Egger, Champion & Bolton, 1998).

Weight machines are preferable for the elderly because:

- Weight machines take away the problem of balance which is an added risk both for the participant and trainer.

- The use of seating and belts creates an added protection for the lower back.

- Handles for gripping are an added advantage taking into consideration that blood pressure can be elevated by excessive gripping.

- Low level weights to start with eliminate risks for new elderly participants.

- However, weights can be increased in small components allowing for challenges especially after a plateau effect. (Egger, Champion & Bolton, 1998).

**All-Purpose Guidelines:**

A warm-up needs to be performed before any exercise and flexibility is increased by a thorough stretching session. Motivation is an important aspect of getting elder people to undertake exercise and emphasis should be placed on body weight, movement and quality of life. Supervised sessions should allow for a slow build up of resistance weights and competency.

Regular workouts should be encouraged – so that the gains can be experience and the habit instilled. Even though the commencement might be slow – considerable gains can be made in strength using weights frequently.

Both client and instructor can be rewarded quickly with strength training but it is important to keep the benefits flowing evenly and not allowing the client to do excessive exercise which may be tiring or damaging to joints and muscles.

## Women and Resistance Training

Women have a more reduced cross-section area in each muscle fibre than men and their muscles yield less tension per unit volume. This makes it much more difficult to develop the muscle size and capacity of men especially since women produce a tenth of the testosterone that men do.

Instead of affecting the contractile structures of their muscles, women have the capacity to efficiently recruit the motor nerves. This means that women can develop strength to the same degree as men potentially.

Women can achieve strength in the hips and legs to a greater degree than men but rarely take up the opportunity to develop the same muscle weight as men.

## Exercise Programming and Relevant Factors

Even if exercise is minimal it can produce some solid benefits and help to retain a basis fitness mode. Among the most significant profits are:

- The ageing effect is postponed in the physiological body

- Coronary heart disease risks are diminished

- Self-confidence rises, stress is reduce and there are further psychological benefits associated with well-being

- Respiratory and cardiovascular effectiveness is increased

- Less risk of metabolic diseases such as obesity, diabetes, lipidaemia.

For people over fifty, physical fitness can enhance strength, flexibility, muscle endurance, cardiovascular (heart/lung) productivity as well as the most important aspects of balance and agility.

Mobility itself, becomes a challenge for older people and as a result – lifestyle options can be severely limited. Any fitness program should be designed to take into consideration client needs of stamina, suppleness, strength and speed. One problem for example for many older people is muscle and joint stiffness whereby a flexibility program would help a great deal in mobility, reflex ability and confidence to engage in a range of activities. Motivation can come from the trainer or instructor but the client will have to find even better reasons for changing a sedentary lifestyle. Most trainers would advocate at least three training sessions a week, but why not every day? Why not several sessions a day? The revolutionary step is to prioritise exercise so that it leads the client's lifestyle and other things fit around it. This is not an obsessive activity but rather one of knowledge and commitment – expecting the best results and influencing peers to also follow a good example. When St. Benedict founded his religious order if the fifth century A.D., he designed a social model built around prayer every hour and integrated then with intellectual and manual work. This was to avoid social chaos following the fall of Rome. Today we are facing a similar crisis brought about by inactivity, immobility, obesity and yet experiencing longevity.

## Principles of Exercise Prescription to Bring About Change:

### Age and Adaptation:

In the early stages of an exercise program, the untrained person can expect some rewarding changes. However, if the client is already in an exercise program, changes and gains need to be made through 'smart' training and age will be a factor for this adaptation as well as genetic potential.

### Warm-up:

If the client engages in any competitive sport as well as being a general principle, warm-ups boost performance and lessen the risk of injury. They also provide a space for psychological preparation of strategies. There will be an acceleration of blood flow the muscles and tissues and body temperature will increase 1-2 degrees as the heart rate increases – nutrients are carried to the contracting muscles and oxygen assists in the elimination of lactic acid wastes and carbon dioxide.

As the muscles warm up, contractions can increase in rate and force while injury risk is reduced by suppleness of connective tissues. As the Central Nervous System becomes involved – a host of reactions, co-ordination and skills are informed.

The Central Nervous System is informed by a warm up particularly if movement patterns are selected which match the exercise about to be performed. During the warmup – repetitious movement raises the body temperature the targeted muscle groups assist in shifting blood to the arterioles of those selected areas.

**Cool-down:**

During the cooling off process – the body returns to the physiological resting state. With a steady reduction in the intensity of exercise, blood returns to the heart and is not pooled in the limbs.

**Why Stretch?**

- **To Help Prevent Injuries.** When muscles change in length or meet with unpredictable energy, there is a need for flexibility. Lack of flexibility can mean damaging a muscle and not being able to perform a range of functions which can also have serious consequences.
- **To Decrease Delayed Onset Muscle Soreness (DOMS).** Without stretching, muscles can experience a range of unanticipated actions which will cause delayed onset muscle soreness (DOMS).
- **To Promote Good Mobility of the Joints.** Ligament stretching is as important as muscle stretching and it enhances the movement of the joints overall. Joints need to reach a full range of motion, be flexible and to relax.
- **To Help Posture and Back Pain.** The tightening of support muscles in the lower back and pelvis can result in back pain as well as altering posture.
- **Tension and Stress Can be Reduced** Stress is often the cause of taut muscles in the shoulders and neck resultant in headaches. Anxiety, tension and other effects of stress can be greatly assisted by stretching.

**How to Stretch:**

Stretches should avoid bounce and be perfectly static – performed with a moderate, slow flow and held for 15-20 seconds. It is also important to experience tension within the muscle set.

**When to Stretch:**

A gentle warmup before a stretch will ensure a lower risk of injury. The temperature of the body will rise and overall levels out the intensity of the exercise session in the cooling down process. This progressive formula manages to keep muscles relaxed throughout the session.

**Training for Aerobic Fitness**

**Frequency:**

Walking is excellent incidental exercise and assists with continuity of mobility, gait posture and well-being. However to develop aerobic fitness requires the heart rate to reach 60-80% of its maximal effort through aerobic fitness exertion of 20-60 minutes, although walking may create this effect in an obese person.

**Overload:**

Training at a higher level than the individual comfort zone, the muscles increase in strength and achieve a higher level of cardiorespiratory fitness. The fitness level is raised as the physical body adapts to meet the training threshold. Muscles enjoy surprise and stimulation rather than a repetition of the same type and at the same level.

**Specificity:**

Targeting special muscle groups or levels of fitness require precise exercises. It is important for the training program put forward to match the goals and to satisfy all expectations rather than to generalise and risk disappointment and abandonment of program.

**Reversibility:**

Commitment to a program and its prioritisation in the life of the client can make the difference between continuity and dropping out when the going gets tough or repetitive. An estimate of 6 weeks in discontinuity can mean the loss of benefits from the exercise program or a similar loss of intensity in the training program can affect advancement.

### Individuality:

One size or exercise prescription does not fit all people. A program should demonstrate a response to individual needs as well as taking into account injury contraindications and specific training goals and potentiality. The individual's specific training history will also be taken into account.

### Recovery:

Once in full exercise mode, many people find it difficult to take recovery seriously as they forge ahead with the next set or training exercises. However rest is needed within and between muscle groups and body parts and time out to break down lactic acid deposits. For example, a serious weight lifter will develop training towards shorter sessions which are more intense but governed by longer periods between working out so that the body fully recovers from its physical exertion

### Periodisation:

Periodisation is a method of training which breaks the program up into defined periods of time, each period having a specific goal. The parameters of fitness focused on in each period will be different. This a particularly useful way of training for an event such as a mini marathon or a sporting event which is some months away. Each week of that period will be planned setting different goals, intensity of training and varied recovery periods. The objective will also be to reach a peak before the event to allow for some recovery and not to be too exhausted on the big day.

### Progression:

Continued progression comes from increasing intensity and duration of exercise sessions and can be built into program planning. One of the most common mistakes in exercise, is the repetition of training programs which leave the mind and muscles thoroughly untested.

## CHAPTER FOUR:  Cardiorespiratory Training

Choosing the best equipment in a gym setting for mature-aged cardiorespiratory training involves the efficacy of enhancing power sport skills, strength, increased aerobic fitness and the decrease of body fat as outlined below:

### Exercise Bikes:

Stationery bikes are useful for arthritic or overweight clients and the elderly while increasing leg and joint mobility.   The bike can also be used in confined space in other settings and affords a stable yet aerobic component.   Bikes are also practical for warming up and cooling down activities.

### Treadmills:

As well as indoor stationary cycling,  the basic treadmill  offers the opportunity of indoor walking and jogging on a treadmill.  Especially in unseasonal weather conditions, the treadmill experience burns up body fat and again is useful for a warm up or cool down.

### Rowing Machines:

Upper body workouts which are more effective than cycling or running on a treadmill can be achieved through a rowing machine.

### Skipping ropes:

Although useful as a fitness tool, research has demonstrated that there are no direct benefits in terms of increased heart rate and muscle involvement, above jogging.


## PLANNING A CIRCUIT:

### Circuits using Free Weights, Machines and Equipment:

To mix machine and equipment use with free weights for an older population, a circuit can be planned using the following exercises:

- Exercise Bike
- Pullovers
- Lunges
- Dumbbell Flyers
- Abdominal Crunch
- Power Clean
- Mini Trampoline
- Upright Row
- Abdominal Crunch
- Press Behind Neck
- Skipping
- Squats
- Bench Press
- Abdominal Crunch
- Power Clean
- Mini trampoline
- Upright Row
- Bicep Curl
- Exercise Bike

## Machine System Equipment Circuit:

Rather than mixing machines with non-equipment circuits, divisions can be made between the two methods. A further selection can then be utilised within the equipment-based circuit of the use of equipment with hydraulic cylinders and machines equipped with cams and cables.

## Non-Equipment Circuits:

These circuits without equipment bring variation and an element of fun to exercise which will be appreciated by mature participants as well as younger clients and they are excellent substitutes for an aerobic class which might be more physically taxing in that there is often no break between movements.

- Side leg lifts (right side)
- Dips Squats with lateral raise

- Push-ups with hands wide
- Tuck jumps
- Abdominal crunch
- Forward lunge (alternate legs)
- Side leg lifts (left side)
- Push-ups with hands close
- Reverse curl
- Free squats
- Karate punches
- Reverse lunge (alternative legs)
- Step ups

**Guidelines for Aerobic Exercise Programs:**

Genuine aerobic activities work the heart and lungs as well as the limbs but there is always caution in relation to age, any medical conditions and fitness levels. Nevertheless, aerobic exercise can be enjoyable and challenging to mature age groups and includes swimming, jogging, cycling, dancing, running and skipping. Within the gym, aerobic activity is created through treadmills, exercise bikes, circuit trainers, steppers and aerobic classes which usually incorporate co-ordinated dance movements. This type of co-ordination can be very beneficial for the over fifties in achieving balance, co-ordination and sequence skills – in other words a genuine 'high' occurs here!

In creating aerobic exercise programs it is valuable to create standards such as the following:

- Encourage your clients to exercise regularly and three times weekly should be a minimum.
- Stretching over a full range of motion for a short period combined with a warmup at the beginning of the program is important. At the end of the aerobic class, cool down with slow static stretching. Each component of stretching, warmup and aerobic exercise as well as the cool-down – should be gradual.
- Where possible, avoid bouncy (ballistic) movements which may occur more frequently with inexperienced exercisers.

- Most aerobic classes are conducted for levels of experience (and fitness) with beginners and advanced clients being separated. In older groups this may not be such an issue as it would not be common to find advanced exercisers. However, in future years this could all change.

- Any new class participants should be screened for their level of exercise and fitness and placed in a class which is appropriate.

- With specific exercises and procedures, it is important to make sure that participants can execute them properly without causing stress and duress to the muscular and joint functions.

- A minimum heart rate of 120bpm creates an intensity measure which provides a genuine aerobic workout over a period of approximately 20 minutes.

- Women will have more flexibility with adductor/abductor and back stretches than men and letting clients know the levels of difficulty that might be encountered in the aerobic activity can avoid drop-outs and injury.

- Advise older clients on clothing to prevent overheating and enhance comfort particularly if they have little exercise experience.

- Any accompanying music with an aerobics classes should provide a beat for slow warm-ups, stretches and cool-downs of up to 5 minutes each.

- Precautions must be taken at all times to prevent both acute and chronic injury. This includes the overuse of certain techniques such as bouncing on toes, or running with bare feet on hard surfaces.

- There should not be any surprises for an older population - let participants know the length of the aerobic program and any different aspects that may occur during the exercises.

- Participants must be asked if they are taking any form of medication, and if so, what this may be. Where no knowledge about a medication is immediately available, steps should be taken to ascertain contraindications, if any.

- Limited non-alcoholic intake and exercise should be before meals rather than after. If an exercise program is prolonged, it might be advisable to take fluids during the aerobic activity.

- Dehydration is another factor which can

- affect older clients whether exercising or not.
- Appropriately cushioned shoes will bring comfort and prevent injury for mature clients especially for running, skipping and balance such as in hopping.
- Again, warm-ups are imperative before joining the aerobics class.

## CHAPTER FIVE: Energy Systems

## ATP:

ATP or adenosine triphosphate is the energy created from the breakdown of food. The makeup is a sugar molecule (adenosine) and three phosphate groups. Higher energy bonds are formed by the chemical bonds between the terminal phosphate groups. Energy is freed when the bond is broken during a chemical reaction and the sliding filaments in the myofibrils are activated allowing for muscle contraction.

## Sources of ATP:

There are three different pathways and energy processes by which ATP might be replenished once its limited quantity has been broken down in the muscle cells and requires regeneration.

1. The ATP/PC or phosphagen system allows for the resynthesis of ATP from the breakdown of phosphcreatine (PC).

2. Anaerobic glycolysis or the lactic acid system - the partial breakdown of glucose or glycogen carbohydrates (CHO) enables the resynthesis of ATP and the creation of energy.

3. The aerobic or Oxygen (02) system. CHO, protein and fats are broken down completely to create the energy for the re-synthesis for ATP.

The reconstitution of ATP molecules from the release of energy of the breakdown of PC, CHO, proteins and fats all work in a similar way. The actual couple reactions are simultaneous catabolic and anabolic reactions.

## The Anaerobic System:

ATP is replenished by the partial breakdown of glucose or glycogen during anaerobic glycolysis or the lactic acid system process. The phosphate system and the lactate system are two very different routes of energy production. The phosphate system is able to provide energy immediately from the resources of the muscles while the lactate system depends on food sources in the absence of oxygen.

### The Lactate System:

Although we don't envisage people over 50 and 60 and older going into major swimming or running events – some do and it important to know how the Lactic Acid System becomes the foremost supplier of ATP for high power events. These events could be a 400 metre run lasting 10-60 seconds or say a 200 metre swim. Pyruvic acid forms ATP when the fuel of carbohydrates assists in the breakdown of glycogen in the muscles. When there is no oxygen, glycogen is only partly broken down and the resulting lactic acid causes muscle fatigue.

### The Phosphate System:

When muscle contractions are repeated, ATP must be reloaded instantly. Phosphocreatine is broken down without the assistance of oxygen and both ATP and Phosphocreatine are found in very small amounts within the muscles (about 85 grams). When the body cannot break down glycogen quickly to form ATP, the ATP-PC system takes over. However, the ATP source in the skeletal muscles can be depleted after a fifteen to twenty second exertion at a maximal effort. When activities are longer, ATP must be resynthesised from other energy bases.

Duration and intensity in exercise will alter the rates of interchange and overlap between these energy systems:

- The phosphate system is engaged when a single movement of about 1 second is executed.

- A short sprint of 10 seconds involves the phosphate system.

- The phosphate/lactate systems can be engaged with a strong 10-60 second sprint.

- The lactate/aerobic systems come on board with a mid-distance sprint of about 1-6 minutes.

- Aerobic energy is used during a 2 hour marathon event or longer.

Phosphate/lactate and aerobic energy systems will be employed during floor classes, extended circuit training and team games which last more than 1 hour.

**The Aerobic System:**

Of all the energy systems, the aerobic system produces more energy when large amounts of oxygen are transported to the muscles as energy, and exercise is increased. The muscle cells contain mitochondria where the lactic acid, carbohydrate fats and protein are broken down. When a person's maximum capacity for consuming oxygen is measured – the related aerobic capacity can be measured (VO2max). It is the efficiency of the cardiovascular system in transporting oxygen to the cells which determines a person's aerobic fitness. The ways in which this can be upgraded are:

- If you increase an exercise or activity by 20-30 minutes there will be an upgraded fitness effect.

- Aerobic energy systems are improved by the full utilisation of shoulders, trunk, thighs and arms.

- A guide to greater aerobic fitness would be an increment of the heart rate to more than 120 beats per minute.

Recovery requires the cessation of activity for a period of one hour, one day or a longer period depending upon the work undertaken. This allows for the replenishment of the energy store that was exhausted. Accumulated lactic acid in the muscles and blood also needs to be removed so that the body recovers to a pre-exercise capacity

**Aerobic/anaerobic Threshholds:**

It is necessary to know when the body is approaching a threshhold to understand the onsets between the energy systems and why the accumulated lactic acid causes discomfort. If you take a run with different pacing, such as steady, sprints, hills, it is possible to engage each of the energy systems described above.

Intensity in any activity will increase the heart rate and roughly 130 beats per minute and below characterise aerobic metabolism. There is a moderate increase in ventilation and very little alteration in the blood lactate levels with demonstrated energy intensity.

The maximal oxygen uptake (VO2Max) will be between 40-70% when the heart rate reaches 130-150 beats per minute achieving the aerobic threshold. Although blood lactate levels and ventilation naturally increase – during aerobic activities such as running and swimming – the exercise can be kept up for some hours.

The anaerobic energy pathway is opened when an even higher level of intensity is reached so that it becomes the dominant source of energy but such intensity can only be sustained for a few minutes. The heart rate increases as does ventilation and there is an accumulation of blood lactate. To achieve higher performance levels, athletes aim to intensify their anaerobic thresholds and thus escalate endurance through the aerobic energy system.

Fatigue is apparent when there is a low aerobic/anaerobic threshold and when fitness has been an issue for people over 50 then this most certainly will be experienced. A combination of energy systems is used in the majority of exercises and activities. There is a need for a greater blood supply when large muscle groups are employed. An increased heart rate with an ongoing activity of over 35 minutes will probably overload the aerobic system. High impact movement will demand the transition to the phosphate anaerobic pathway threshold. What is reassuring is that even with older clients, the adoption of a cardiovascular training program will be able to achieve a higher level of fitness through a heightened energy threshold. Most people over fifty, starting exercise for the first time – will attribute their lack of fitness to age rather than their lack of commitment to regular exercise. The first step is to try it out and see how successfully training can change health and lifestyle.

## CHAPTER SIX:    Training for Flexibility & Suppleness

Flexibility is one of the most important aspects of health and fitness in an ageing population.   It is also frequently overlooked and a passive attitude towards mobility and agility exercises can impact severely on body stress levels and flexibility limitations as would ignoring cardiovascular and resistance activities. A flexibility workout will assist posture especially chronic conditions of sway back, flat back and kyphosis/lordosis – rounded shoulders and even a pronounced hump. Many people over fifty (particularly those who have been sitting in an office for years) need to improve mobility and reduce back and neck pain which can be greatly assisted by flexibility workouts.

### Age:

The connective tissue surrounding the muscles and the ligaments attaching joints can also lose elasticity as people age.   The predominantly inactive lifestyle of an older population actually works towards limited mobility.

### Exercise:

When we move, the muscles naturally shorten and contract.   Even continual movement in everyday life, without flexibility work, can lead to residual shortening of muscle tissue and connective ligaments, leaving our bodies feeling stiffer, causing muscular imbalances and reducing the range of movement.

### Joints:

A 'whole' body approach improves flexibility and mobility.   Although flexibility may have been achieved in one part of the body – flexibility in the body is also specific to each joint and its configuration. You may be flexible in one part of your body, but this is not indicative of your overall flexibility levels.   For example arms may be used a great deal more than legs or ankles and sometimes this is governed by the onset of osteoarthritis.   The more painful a joint is to use the more it is neglected. However, even conditions such as osteoarthritis require the ongoing use of the joint to provide the maximum flexibility that is possible under the circumstances.

**The Benefits of Stretching:**

A flexibility and mobility programme:

### 1. Increases the functional range of motion of each joint.

Each joint has a functional range motion and inflexibility in age could prevent the independence of reaching for kitchen objects, bending for tying up shoe laces even having difficulties with dressing, zippers or clasps!

**Reduces lower back pain and risk of injury.**

Back pain is caused by a lack of pelvic flexibility and the imbalance of muscles in the trunk and core body regions. It is also a major disability for both young and old – causing the loss of a huge number of working days and in the aged – the further risk of injury and immobility.

**Decreases the severity of a potential injury.**

If you consider the optimal flexibility in elite athletes, whether in be skiing, diving or team sport – there is reduced state of injury through their flexibility training activities. Older people, particularly over 70 years of age, experience falls which could be prevented in many cases by flexibility training and the building up of certain muscle groups. Falls in an elderly population present one of the most serious hazards to well-being and health, whether people live in their own homes or in an aged care facility.

## CHAPTER SEVEN:  Core Stability Exercises

The torso which contains the thoracic cavity and the abdominal cavity make up the torso.  The stability of this vulnerable area depends upon the ability to resist forces which would  interfere with and destabilise the torso.   The ribs limit the movement of the thoracic vertebrae and act as a cage around the thoracic cavity.

However, the capacity  and function of the lumbar spine is  to be more mobile and less protected as well as carrying extra weight.  The building and reinforcement of the muscles of the abdominal cavity are very important.  These include - posteriorly,  the erector spinae muscle group, the pelvic floor muscles below, the diaphragm above and the abdominal muscles.

**The benefits of core stability for the over fifties:**

- Forms the basis for limbs to produce more force

- There is an improvement in posture

- Especially reduces the risk and event of falls in the elderly

- Considerably heightens prevention and/or rehabilitation of injuries to the spine

To maintain a sustained, co-ordinated contraction of the core and pelvic muscles and achieve core stability, the following are important:

- Selected muscles must be able to adjust quickly to changing loads

- Muscle strength developed  in appropriate muscles

- Endurance of the right muscles

- Feedback about the position of the body and the way in which forces are applied (proprioceptive/kinaesthetic) via the nervous system.

- Muscle group co-ordination.

**Types of core stability exercises:**

The usefulness of core stability exercises is extended to rehabilitation of injuries and is usually done on a fitball (Swiss ball) or on the floor. The musculoskeletal function, posture and movement are all related and to discover the role of strength, stability and flexibility – the fitball or floor exercises serve well as demonstrations.

Once postural analysis and screening are undertaken, weaknesses can be assessed. A strategy is worked out as well as stretches and feedback so that a person can understand how to make changes and use the body appropriately. Training the neuromuscular system using the actual movement pattern creates the most successful approach. Observation by the trainer is important and exercises should not isolated but a whole sequence of movement set in motion.

**Principles of core stability training:**

- Precision and control need to be learnt.

- Transverse Abdominis is the abdominal muscle which should be isolated and other superficial muscles avoided.

- Once control over Transverse Abdominis is mastered there can be an incorporation and contraction of other abdominal muscles.

- Motor learning is the key to stabilising core segments of the body.

- Slow and controlled contractions are the best way to train and utilise the abdominal muscles.

- Core segments of the body are stabilised through a motor learning approach.

- Core stability exercises need to be practised daily.

- The key to success in core stability is the repetition of the contractions and follow through exercises.

# CHAPTER EIGHT:  Outdoor Activity

At least 50% of the body's muscle mass (or more) needs to be involved in aerobic exercise which is associated with cardiovascular endurance. The minimal amount of exercise which allows for a sustained training and aerobic effect will probably not be found in golf or bowls but that doesn't mean that these are not recreational and enjoyable and far better than 'sitting at home'.   Continuous, rhythmic exercise which will produce an aerobic effect could be swimming, running and jogging, dancing and vigorous walking if the FITT formula (frequency, intensity, time and type) is to be followed.   Aerobic exercises also can be individual or groups activities

## Solo Exercise:

In some ways solo exercise is more spiritually uplifting as well as meeting aerobic requirements.  In those beautiful spaces such as a forest way, park, beach and fields, the simple pleasure of being one with the environment and nature  at an aerobic pace can be elevating.  Other people or elaborate equipment are not needed  - just the wind in your hair.  There is a wonderful feeling of independence and control over a person's own exercise program  which can produce  much pleasure as well as a training effect.  Solo work can include cycling, swimming, surfing, jogging, weight training, skipping and some fast forms of aerobic yoga exercises.

In developing cardiovascular fitness, a comparison can be made between running and swimming where there are equal intensities utilised so that there is roughly a ratio of 5:1 or a 5km run to match a 1km swim.

## Instructor-Based Exercise:

Many people prefer social interaction and are more highly motivated when they have a group activity.  Leadership to the activity may also be a key to keeping older people involved in the activity as well as choice of music and the ease of executing the aerobic activity.

Circuit classes can be fun as well as step classes, aquarobics, aerobics and dance classes.

A longer session of swimming, jogging or cycling might elevate the heart rates to 129-140 bpm, for which energy is necessary to run a 10 minute mile pace. In addition, aerobic dancing requires twice as much effort and energy than traditional dancing.

**One-to-One:**

Competitive games often provide more enjoyment, camaraderie, flexibility and co-ordination skills. Competitors should be equally capable and skilled to have continuous dual activity. Activities in this category are tennis, boxing, badminton and squash.

Advanced fitness levels require the selection of sports and activities with greater overloads such as squash, handball and badminton but beginners might select a sport like singles tennis to improve initial fitness. So racquet sports are not all even in their deliverance of aerobic fitness – rather they provide a graded selection for each level of fitness and competency.

**Team Games:**

Among the greatest combinations of social and fitness goals are team sports and competition adds to the excitement and stimulation. Touch football, cricket, water polo, softball, surf lifesaving, volleyball and netball are among the many team games which provide these excellent fitness combinations.

Anaerobic or phosphate energy systems are used in stop-go actions so that aerobic conditioning is not constantly engaged such as in the continuous movement of soccer, hockey, water polo or basketball.

**Getting Away:**

Three times a week is considered the minimum commitment to any fitness-enhancing activity to achieve the desired levels. Although many of these activities would defy the capacity and skills of older people, some will have gained them during more youthful times and continue to practice them – for example mountain climbing, rowing, canoeing, skiing and orienteering. Bush walking is for all ages and one of the most stimulating and energising activities of later age. Getting away for a few days is a wonderful way for an aged population to stay fit and to be stimulated by new surroundings.

## Swimming:

For people over fifty and every decade onwards, swimming is the key to staying fit when risky impacts might prevent taking up other activities. Swimming is a particularly effective and therapeutic form of activity if a person suffers from osteoarthritis or rheumatoid arthritis. If the client is not a swimmer, aqua aerobics can be a successful alternative and is a wonderful exercise for rehabilitating injuries to the body. The body is given buoyancy and support and joint pain is alleviated during exercise.

## Running:

Running is successful in burning more calories than other activities. For older people, an alternation between walking and jogging might be a more successful way to begin. When the cardiovascular fitness has been improved, running can be attempted slowly. It is important to avoid running on hard surfaces where the impact may cause wear and tear on the spine.

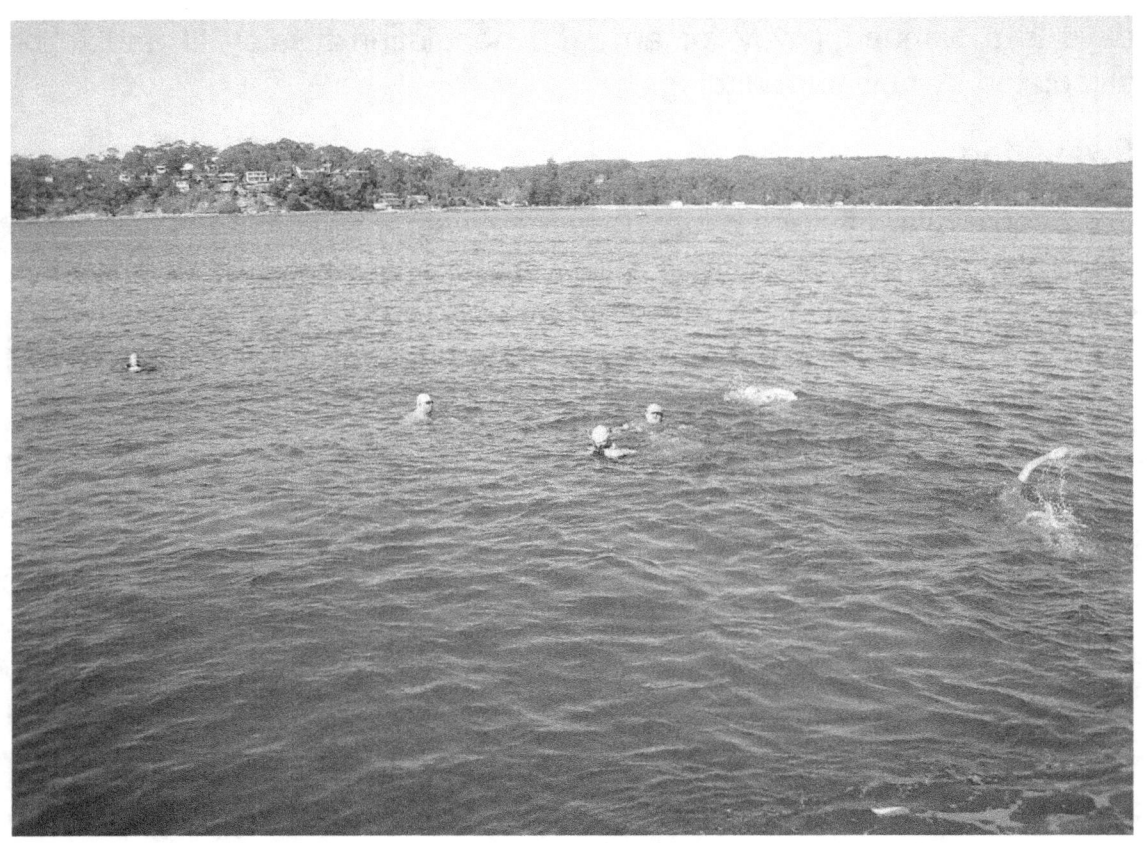

I live near the coast so I generally swim along a bay beach, about 600 metres most mornings, just taking it really easy.

I've been swimming since I was a kid and enjoy swimming in the sea best but in past years when I've lived away from the coast swimming in the local pool has been OK.

A while ago I was having some painful shoulder problems and the physiotherapist I visited gave me some exercises pulling my hand forward using a theraband. I get really bored with such exercises and after talking with my physiotherapist - we worked out that swimming backstroke would give me essentially the same exercise. I'd always swum overarm before so it took me a while to get used to backstroke with lots of mouthfuls of water and coughing. But after a while it all came together and now it's a great pleasure to look up at the beautiful cloud formations while I'm swimming. From time to time the terns circle looking for small fish just below the surface. When one is spotted, the tern goes into a steep dive to plunge into the water. It's a pleasure to watch nature working like this. I sometimes think they might dive on me but I don't think they're the least bit interested – I'm not food!

Swimming for pleasure is quite easy to learn. I know of a number of people around my age who have taken it up in earnest not having swum much before. The key is a good instructor to point you in the right direction for breathing and stroke. It's just practice after that.

I generally swim through the winter when the water temperature gets down to 17 degrees or less, although not as frequently. I find that a wetsuit designed for swimming keeps me warm quite well. When I do swim in the winter, and often in the summer, it's with a number of like-minded friends. It's easier getting into the water on a cold day when you're with others rather than doing it alone. After our swim, we usually go to a local café for a nice hot coffee. It feels really great.

David Gosden

**PART TWO:  Exercise for Special Groups**

**CHAPTER NINE:  Identifying specific population client basis.**

**Clients with Disability:**

Disability referrals and their identification may come from allied health professionals, medical practitioners and workers' compensation professionals.  Often the referral will identify a need but the referrer is not necessarily trained in a therapeutic approach to all of the rehabilitation needs to be identified in clients with a disability. The clients could then belong to any age group and be part of a client base already.

By networking through medical practitioners, insurance groups dealing in workplace injury compensation, workers' compensation listings and allied health professionals who specialise in disability population support and welfare, client bases and marketing strategies are worked out for specific populations.  There also needs to be differentiation in publicizing the program to distinct categories of age and gender within the disability population range itself.

Determination of the fitness service requirements of a specific disability group will also need to look at the facilities, geographical area and target area in marketing.  The range of facilities and services might include targeting gentle exercise, resistance training, water exercise and sports, exercise style and intensity, specific equipment and a range of disability-friendly facility environments.

In planning a fitness program, all other additional health problems must be considered.  A supervising medical or health professional may have specific requirements associated with the client's rehabilitation and injury.

In designing a marketing program for specific population client groups with disability, the legal rights of the disability population should be considered including visual graphics, text and language to generate empathy and consideration to potential clients.   Professionals should also be familiar with equal opportunity legislation and anti-discrimination legislation.

Exercise delivery for a disability client base might require resources such as wheelchair access and perhaps referrals from a speech therapist. Exercise professionals could benefit from marketing tools such as Morgan Surveys in order to locate demographics of a specific population. The use of questionnaires, clinics, telephone marketing and hospitals, nursing homes and consultation with potential clients could be fruitful. A further aspect of business marketing and care and communication with the client, would be the establishment of supporting relationships with appropriate stakeholders, such as relatives, clinics, hospitals and general practitioners.

These chapters explore the role and application of exercise prescription in the management of specific aged clients and those with chronic health conditions. When looking at cardiovascular, respiratory, metabolic and musculoskeletal disorders, along with their risk factors of secondary disease – exercise tolerance and functional status is considered. Fundamental concepts in exercise testing and programming to enhance physical health and those with cognitive impairments are also observed.

## CHAPTER TEN:  Consultative Networks:  exercise physiologists and trainers, allied health and medical advisers.

Consultative networks of professionals might include the assessment, prescription of exercise for clients with injury or disease in relation to rehabilitation and prevention by exercise scientists.  A more direct role would be played by physiotherapists, osteopaths and occupational therapists in specifying what the exercise program should accomplish. Trainers and sports coaches may have a more limited role and counsellors may prescribe exercise to people suffering emotional needs and motivation deficits associated with depression, just as psychologists address mental health problems frequently by directing their clients to outdoor exercise.  The musculoskeletal therapist - osteopaths and physiotherapist focus on rehabilitation for injury while massage therapists might identify complex skeletal maladjustments and tight muscle areas and those therapists direct their clients to exercise programs.

When a client experiences depression, joint and back pain, obesity, headaches and overall lack of fitness, a general practitioner would possibly request an assessment of fitness and refer the client to an exercise program.  Psychiatrists might want to address bipolar and severe mental health problems, whereas a medical specialist might be focussing upon a special problem within the musculoskeletal spectrum. Exercise programs are often also prescribed by clinical nurse consultants for mental health clients as well as referring patients with physical disabilities and health needs.  To maintain this consultative network, exercise therapists should be able to create a proposal for the specific group and ask for consultation with medical and allied health professionals to be able to provide feedback on the efficacy and benefits of the program.

Communication with the aged may have its own special challenges such as visual impairment or hearing loss.  It is important that clients can fully understand and interpret instructions in regard to achieving the exercise goal and also safety.

Local council activities, rehabilitation clinics, seniors groups, church groups should also be canvassed for potential specific client populations. Again Weightwatchers could provide many interested and dedicated clients who would work in tandem with Weightwatchers' philosophy and an exercise program to reach their goals.

Measuring progress for special populations is essential and baseline performance needs to be set and progress measured with follow-up assessments. Motivation can be a challenge for specific populations and older clients, so goal setting should include a focus on building confidence. Waist/circumference measurements, skinfold and body weight would be included in the assessment protocols while other procedures might gauge changes in performance in physical, psychological or anthropometrical outcomes. If contraindications or limitations are observed then adjustments should be made to the program.

In choosing the type of exercise selection and functional capacity, there may be clinical concerns concerning a disability and disease state. The type of exercise and choice of intensity will also be guided by this criteria as well as contra-indications and risks. Equipment modification is another outcome of monitoring and assessment, and extra assistance might be needed for moving the client on or off equipment and providing handrails for some aged or disability clients.

# CHAPTER ELEVEN: Motivation Theory and Practical Techniques

In working with specific populations it is most important to provide clinically significant improvements and a selection of exercises that match client needs. When an exercise regime is endorsed by an allied health professional it is considered essential to explain the purpose and goal of the exercise so that it gains in stature to the client and also motivates them to achieve.

Choosing the right equipment and sequence of exercises are part of addressing correct technique and safety principles in general training and may require modifications in exercise regimes. This will advance safety and efficiency and can be integrated when instructing the client.

The delivery of instructions in a well modulated voice, timing and tempo of accompanying music will also make a difference in client adherence to the regime. A trainer's communication should be rhythmic and well projected to engage the clients and motivate them.

A client will gain self-confidence when instructions reinforce positioning and cueing so that mistakes aren't made. Special client groups are encouraged by the trainer's questioning and listening skills to gauge feedback and the trainer can become skilful in eye contact, facial expressions and body gestures to motivate and direct clients.

When a trainer involves the client, step-by-step in the planning process, there are great motivational advantages. When techniques are applied to aerobic activities which improve self-efficacy and the pleasure principle, the trainer and client can expect greater efficacy. Some trainers achieve behavioural changes by involving family members to join the exercise session and find that the client has a strong motivation to achieve their goal.

Obesity predictors can include lifelong physical inactivity, how the family regard physical exercise and the regular diet of the family. This is where food diaries become useful to track daily intakes of food and fluid and any changes and improvements. This can be accompanied by tracking physical exercise as well and recording type and frequency. By doing this the client can see how to avoid obstacles and where the real problems lie in their goal of weight loss.

One popular and well supported theory for motivation is the 'Health Belief Model' and is explained by the obvious benefits of regular physical activity (weights/training and aerobic exercise) and the association of low cost. The goal of a fat-free mass (skeletal muscles), postural strength and bone mass could encourage clients experiencing obesity while functional capacity is an obvious target for the aged or clients with disability. Increased independence comes from a fully functioning immune system and this is boosted by exercise – maintaining a high level of health and preventing disease of a degenerative nature. Support for the special population client exercise group emerges in the form of increased networks and communal contacts. This works especially well for clients who have depressive illnesses or experience social isolation. Professional medical treatment can be costly and taking on an exercise program and maintaining it, will require only time and energy by comparison.

Varying client cohorts, different environments and specific populations would require different and specific evaluations in regard to motivational theory. The specific populations might vary from hypertensive clients, obese clients to the frail and elderly, or to those with a disability. The experienced and wise instructor will be enthusiastic in the use of feedback – not critical and be responsible for using the feedback as a motivational tool.

For a client suffering from hypertension, the trainer could write up the following plan for example:

1. First of all what medication is the client taking? High impact exercises should not be used and heart rate should not be more than 70% keeping an eye on the intensity and duration of the exercise. When taking on resistance exercise no weights should be used above the head (valsalva manouvre).

2. Aerobic fitness should be increased while dietary fat, alcohol and sodium are to be lowered. The resting heart rate should be decreased while body fat and medication can be reduced.

3. Referrals might come from a lipids clinic, a dietician or a nutritionist. However, it is worth getting a General Practitioners's

medical clearance letter outlining medication limitations if that is an issue.

4. The reduction of high blood pressure and the increase of cardiovascular fitness would be through aerobic training but with no high impact. A wholistic approach would also include progressive resistance training with a variety of exercises to include endurance and strength.

5. Pinplates and arm plates can help to adjust weight lifting equipment.

6. Cardiovascular improvements are the foremost goal for improvement and motivation can be enhanced by using a behavioural contract and reward system. Clients should provide feedback which can then be used for monitoring progress.

7. Make sure the exercise is culturally appropriate and also suits the age and gender of the client.

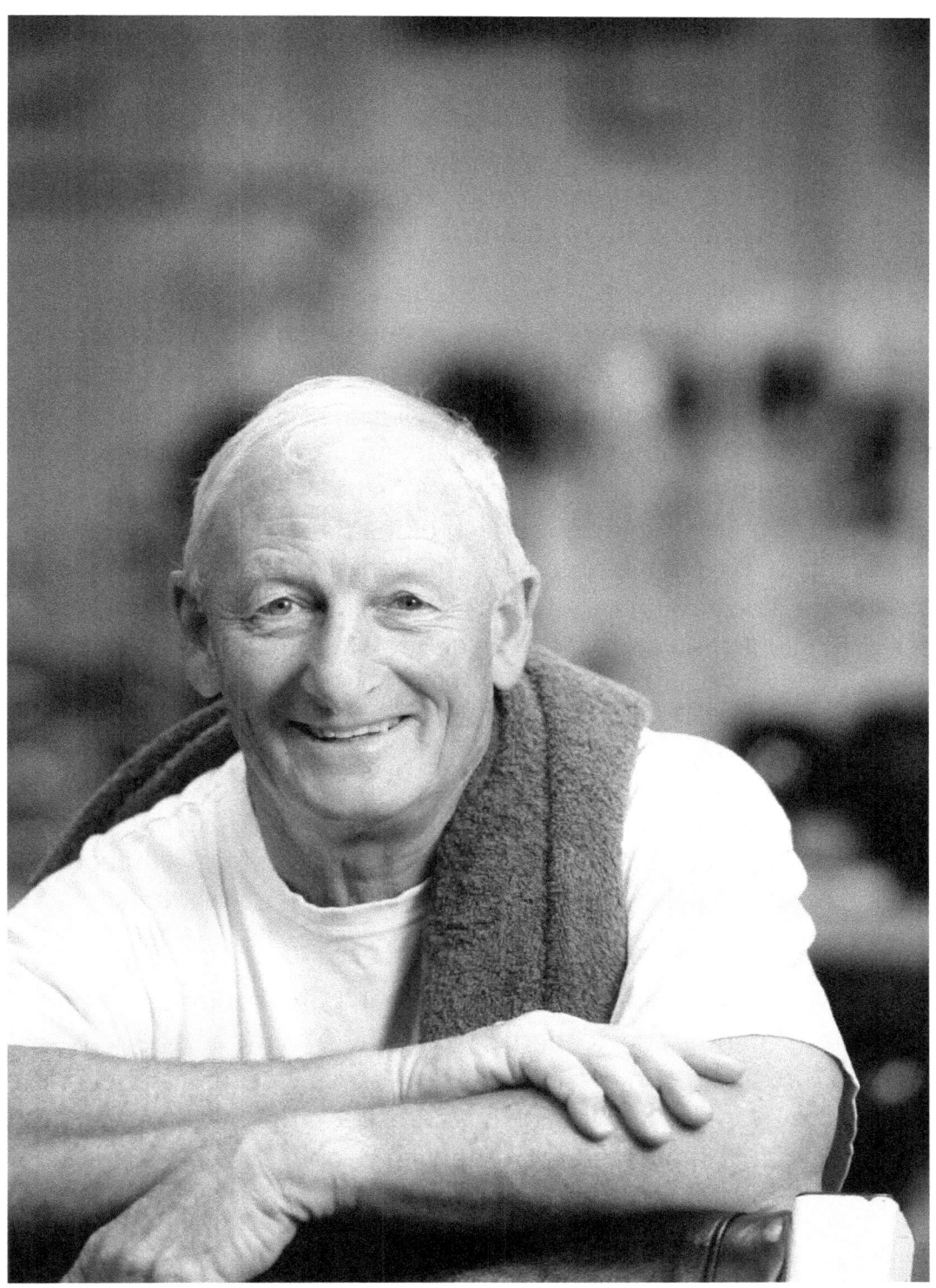

I received an enrolment into a Personal Training Certification for my 70th birthday from my children and combined the training with earlier fitness knowledge to initiate classes for fellow seniors at the University of Sydney Sport & Fitness venue. I've had a very active life as a farmer, builder and business man – and in 1961 toured South Africa as a member of the Wallabies Rugby team.

At Sydney University Sport & Fitness we have large circuit groups for strength training of seniors 60-80 years of age which is also open to local community members. Our numbers can swell to 40 per session, but ideally 25-30 is a maximum. We use all free weights and plenty of core exercises to strengthen the abdominal area, which is important for older people and helps with balance and posture. The circuit goes for about 40 minutes with a minute on each of the 34 stations so that every muscle group is used in the process. The benefits for maintenance of health are great according to feedback and then there is the social aspect, with clients heading off for coffee together after the session.

I've also set up classes for the Bradfield Wellbeing Centre at North Sydney and this caters for clients with mental health problems as well as carers, again attendance continues to rise and clients have reported excellent improvements in all aspects of mental health. I've had the opportunity to introduce exercise in aged care facilities and although this is challenging, the results for mobility and motivation of residents has been very positive.

At 78 my own health is fantastic – rarely a visit to the doctor and I enjoy swimming laps at the Bondi Icebergs Clubs and a round of golf at the NSW Golf Club. I can see myself running fitness classes at least until I'm 80 – and may be longer! I think my age allows me to relate well to the seniors and fulfils my passion for helping people and seeing genuine health benefit changes in their lives.

**John 'Sparrow' Dowse**

## CHAPTER TWELVE: Planning an exercise program for a specific client group:

Psychological assessment and physical assessment can be undertaken through the PAR-Q and the needs analysis will also provide the trainer with the client's specific goals. Weight can vary over a 24 hour period and may fluctuate up to 1-2 kilos – so standardising weight can be an important assessment.

If there are limitations to exercise selection it will come out of the physiological, psychological and general health status of the client. The needs analysis and goals acknowledged may include the following selections:

- Weight training and Aerobics

- Gentle Exercise

- Community fitness classes

- Weights training

General fitness goals could be accompanied by disease prevention and treatment of the condition.

General training principles should guide the sequence and order of exercise beginning with warm-up, stretching and progressive increases for endurance and intensity. The time spent on the exercise regime will be matched with the volume required and agreed upon by the trainer and the client which might also be influenced by social and financial constraints. Especially with special population groups, safety and suitability of equipment is essential.

There are enormous social and psychological benefits for older adults in taking up an exercise and fitness regime including:

- Increased social and recreational activities

- Improved self-esteem and self-confidence

- Changed perception of risk

- Maintenance of independent living

- Support and social network increased

Improvement in anthropometrical and physiological health benefits such as:

- Immune system enhanced

- Bone mass increase

- Functional capacity – i.e. independence

- Postural strength

- Prevention of degenerative diseases

- Reduction and prevention of falls


Even in older clients, muscle mass can increase and be observed after several weeks. Before weights training it is advisable for the client to do aerobics and increase strength.

Motivation for older clients will also come from the type of contact and communication provided by the instructor and should involve emails, texts to increase and maintain attendance. Communication should also encourage feedback and together the trainer and client can identify barriers to exercise participation. Social reinforcement can be promoted through understanding age, gender and cultural differences and using feedback in music choices. There is also the opportunity for the trainer to introduce healthy food and fluid selection.

**Rationale and recommendations for a geriatric exercise prescription**

Social, biochemical, psychological and physiological features will comprise the ageing profile and again nutrition intake and fluids must be taken seriously. There may be a recommendation for exercise for any number of age related health conditions, some of the most common being joint replacement, arthritis, hypertension, angina, osteoporosis and intermittent claudication.

Neuromuscular disorders are prevalent in older clients such as Parkinson's disease and stroke while occurrences of metabolic disorders are increasing, for example diabetes, lipidaemia and thyroid disorders. Hearing deficit, anxiety, depression and visual and sensory problems might also be experience by the elderly. Trainers should also be aware of any major surgery that has been experienced such as bypass surgery, joint replacements and surgery for cancer (bowel/prostate/mastectomy).

## CHAPTER THIRTEEN: Exercise Recommendations for an Aging Population

With ageing, comes an increase in adipose mass and augmented truncal and visceral deposition occurs and these changes can be targeted and reduced by resistance and aerobic modalities.

Type 2 (fast twitch) fibres are also diminished as well as skeletal mass with age. Intramuscular fat and connective tissue replace the atrophied muscles.

Another age-related change is decreased bone mass, density and increased bone fragility. Exercise modalities that are recommended include weight-bearing aerobic exercise, resistance training and high impact, high velocity loading of affected skeletal sites. There are obviously strong considerations of counter-effectiveness for joints and other age-related conditions when developing these programs.

Heart rate and blood pressure frequently increases with age but the response to submaximal exercise is a decrease in these conditions. With age also, there may be impaired bar reflex function and postural hypotension in response to stress but this can also be decreased with physical activity. An increase also occurs of total cholesterol and LDL with age and physical exercise demonstrates that this can also be reduced. The nervous system (hormonal and sympathetic), has an increased response to stress with age, and again physical activity can reverse this effectively.

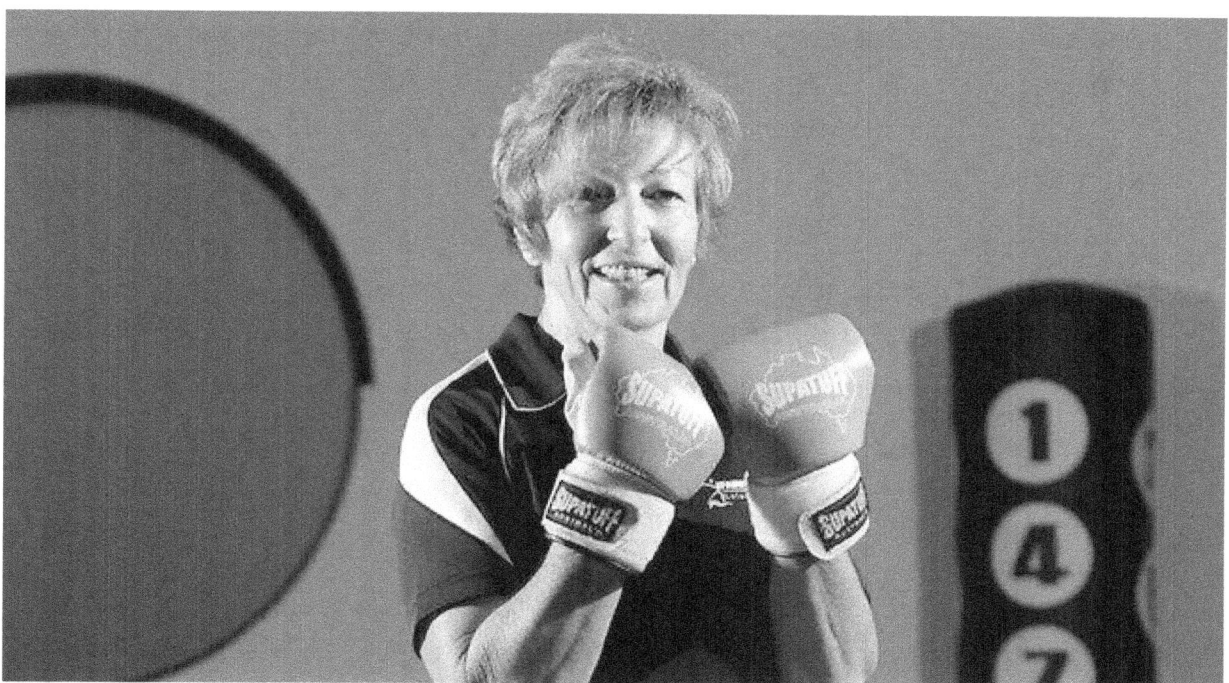

The only exercise I did for many years was walking as the family didn't have a car but after doing office work for many years, I started doing exercising seriously at 39. This became such a passion (and an addiction) that I became a fitness instructor and at 69, I have a very full program as an instructor at three gymnasiums and leisure centres.

I instruct in aerobics, aqua aerobics, boxing for fitness and conduct group personal training and programs for men, women, children and seniors. I also run Pilates and falls prevention classes. I find that the aerobic classes work well for motivating people who find it difficult to exercise alone in the gym. The peer involvement, competition, friendship, mood improvement and stress level reduction are all benefits of aerobics. There is a release of endorphins creating a 'high', while weight reduction and the overall fitness levels increase.

Aqua aerobics works well for people with joint problems through buoyancy and clients have a choice to be in shallow or deep water according to their swimming capacity and joint pain. The class is very relaxing and suits all age groups.

We also using boxing which is a much more intense class – usually working with a partner and suitable for young and middle-aged clients who are reasonably fit and free from injury. A good workout brings 'peace of mind'!

Another favourite is the Pilates class which gives flexibility, strength and conditioning to the clients. It also improves breathing, relaxes the body and brings about a feeling of wellness and inner peace at the completion of the session.

However, personal training is my favourite form of instruction and I tailor programs to suit clients for all reasons including weight loss and fitness/toning.

I'm a veteran of many marathon races but a hip replacement operation made me swap to trekking. My dream was to get to Everest Base Camp and I achieved this two years after the hip replacement operation. It was an emotional and rewarding experience and I continue to trek with my husband and friends in New Zealand, Nepal, Tasmania and other local treks along with power walking.

My own personal fitness provides me with energy to spare - up at 4am, work, exercise and family and keep going until 9pm – and do the same the next day, so although I am 70 next year – I feel 30 years old.

My advice to seniors (over 50) is that you are never too old to exercise. Mobility, strength and fitness are needed for every day life. Incidental exercise, fitness centres, bowling clubs, tennis and other sports are available as well as walking, community clubs and council programs. Any form of exercise can put a smile on your face and promote a healthier and happier life.

**Ann Cusack (Seniors' Week Ambassador 2013)**

## CHAPTER FOURTEEN: Exercise recommendations for prevention, treatment of disease and optimal ageing

**Balance training:** This can be undertaken 1-7 days/wk. The volume should be 10 sets of 4-10 different exercises emphasizing dynamic postures (proprioceptive neuromuscular facilitation involves stretching as far as possible, then relaxing the involved muscles, then attempting to stretch further, and finally holding the maximal stretch position for at least 20 seconds).

Examples of balance enhancing activities include T'ai Chi movements, standing yoga or ballet movements, tandem walking, standing on one leg, stepping over objects, climbing up and down steps slowly, turning, standing on heels and toes, walking on a non-compliant surface such as foam mattresses or sand and maintaining balance on moving a vehicle such as bus or train, etc.

Intensity is increased by decreasing the base of support (e.g. progressing from standing on two feet while holding onto the back of a chair to standing on one foot with no hand support): by decreasing other sensory input (e.g. closing eyes or standing on a foam pillow): or by altering the centre of mass (e.g. holding a heavy object out to one side while maintaining balance, standing on one leg while lifting the other leg out behind body, or leaning forward as far as possible without falling or moving feet).

**Flexibility training:** The frequency of flexibility training can again be 1-7 days a week. The major muscle groups are engaged and there should be a sustained stretch (20 seconds) of each. The intensity reflects the progressive neuromuscular facilitation technique stretching as far as possible, then relaxing the involved muscles – with a final attempt to stretch further and hold that maximal stretch position for at least 20 seconds. For maximal efficiency and safety, static rather than ballistic stretching is recommended.

**Cardiovascular Endurance Training:** This should be undertaken 3-7 days a week for a duration of 20-60 minutes per session. For intensity, the requirement is 12-13 on the Borg Scale (40-60% heart rate reserve or maximal exercise capacity). To maximise effiency and to employ safety requirements, training should be low-impact and weight-bearing if possible and may include standing/walking. To maintain relative intensity, the workload can be increased progressively.

**Resistance Training:** Ideally, resistance training can be implemented 2-3 days a week and volumes of 1-3 sets of 8-12 repetitions for 8-10 muscle groups can be part of the exercise plan. An intensity of 15-17 on the Borg Scale (70-80% IRM), 10 sec/repetition, with 1 minute rest between sets. For safety and maximal efficacy, the speed should be slow with no ballistic movements and a scheduled day of rest between sessions. The form should be good with no substitution of muscles and no breath holding (valsalva manoeuvre). The weights can be progressively increased to maintain relative intensity and if equipment is available, power training (high-velocity, high-loading) provides benefits of both increased strength and power.

## Clients with injuries or medical conditions

While it can be assumed that many older clients have medical conditions, it is necessary in the screening process to identify those conditions and to create treatments plans with a number of considerations. In these special populations, the fitness will also take a secondary role to the advice of other allied health and medical professionals who may be treating the condition. A fitness leader may undertake pre-exercise screening and assessment as well as exercise prescription. Modification and monitoring of the exercise program should be on-going while a fitness assessment and evaluation of the program will be also useful for the allied health and medical professionals treating the client. So a fitness leader will work as part of a team under the supervision of allied health professionals where health, injury or other special conditions have been identified.

Exercise considerations for clients with injury, medical or health conditions with special requirements, will make it important to identify the conditions and the potential effects of exercise upon the condition. In recommending activities, contraindications should be well noted.

The potential irregular effects of exercise due to a client's special condition can include: physiological conditions, heart rate, arrhythmia, ECG, blood pressure, respiratory changes and oedema. The biomechanical effects will relate to the client's centre of gravity, joint laxity, postural limitations, reduced strength, mobility and increased risk of falls.

There may also be nutritional needs – the consequences of inadequate diet and hydration are always an issue for the elderly. The irregular psychological effects of exercise may include a reaction to performance decrements, fat gain or loss, attitude to other trainees/trainers as well as depression and anxiety. Other psychological reactions might be behavioural such as excessive competitiveness, intimidation, emotional disorders and the positive effects of social networking and increased support. Pathological guidelines should be provided by an allied health professional.

## CHAPTER FIFTEEN:   Precautions & Guidelines for Clients with Chronic Ailments

Fitness leaders should be aware of the special precautions when planning and implementing an exercise treatment program for a person suffering from a chronic ailment.

### Benefits of Taking Precautions

The precautions to be taken for exercises related to specific diseases and disorders would be similar to those for general exercise programs including 5 minute warm-ups, going through the motions of the exercise to be performed, marching on the spot and calisthenics.  A cool-down can include a slow walk bringing the heart rate down to around 10 to 15 beats higher than the resting heart rate.  Again, stretching after the cool-down will have great benefits.  Clients with medical conditions should not be exposed to the extreme weather conditions and finally make sure the client is drinking plenty of water at all times.

Certain aerobic dance routines and high-impact exercise could jar joints but well-padded shoes will go a long way to reducing the impact.  Try to organise exercise on soft surfaces where possible.

When strength training older clients, another safety measure is to encourage exhalation during the exertion phase of a manoeuvre and inhalation during the other half of the manoeuvre.  You can use elastic therabands or weight machines and no free weights if strength or balance has declined significantly.

### Special Safety Tips

### Coronary Disease or Hyptertension

Studies show that regular aerobic exercise reduces systolic and diastolic blood pressure by about 10mm Hg.  A word of caution though:  if the client's  resting blood pressure exceeds 200/105, there should be no participation in an aerobic exercise session.  The client should check his or her blood pressure with a General Practitioner.

Warming up prevents a sudden rise in blood pressure and  provides the heart muscle with enough oxygen-bearing blood to meet initial demands of exercise. Any sudden, potentially dangerous drop in blood pressure needs to be avoided. Fluid loss from heavy sweating can cause a potentially dangerous drop in blood pressure and increases the danger of possibly risky blood clots. Conversely, cold constricts blood vessels, raising blood pressure and forcing the heart to pump harder. Polluted air reduces the amount of oxygen reaching the heart muscle. High impact exercise is generally strenuous which can cause an excessive rise in blood pressure or place excessive demands on the heart. Straining to lift excessive weight or holding the breath during the exertion phase of the exercise can cause a potentially dangerous rise in blood pressure.

**Clients with coronary disease**

- Keep heart rate well below level when abnormalities appeared on a stress test.

- Don't exercise a client near busy roads.

- Exercise the client with a companion.

- Carry nitroglycerin when the client exercises. Client should take it if chest pain is experienced; client should then see a doctor as soon as possible. (Or take nitroglycerin before workout instead).

**Clients with hypertension**

- Keep the heart rate below 70% of its maximum rate (220 – client's age)

**Clients on beta-blockers**

- Beta-blockers slow the heart rate, so gauge exercise intensity by perceived exertion, not by heart rate method. To stay in a safe range, exercise should feel somewhat hard but should not make breathing or talking difficult.

## Diabetes

With age it becomes harder to maintain stable blood glucose levels. The cells of the body become more resilient to blood glucose and insulin helps to control blood glucose levels. However, there is a risk of late-onset diabetes (Type 2) and regular exercise and physical activity can improve the body's insulin sensitivity. Through glucose regulation the need for diabetic medication can also be reduced

Exercise protects post-menopausal women against diabetes. Studies found that women between the ages of 55 and 69 who exercised regularly were 31% less likely to develop diabetes than those who did not. And if a client exercises moderately or vigorously more than 4 times a week, the news is even better – the risk of diabetes is half that of women who rarely or never exercise at these levels.

To achieve these benefits, a client can spread out the exercise over the day or week, so that busy people don't necessarily have to spend hours in the gym.

By boosting blood flow, warming up partially compensates for the poor circulation in some diabetics. Cooling down prevents sudden, dangerous drops in blood pressure which are particularly likely in diabetics due to impaired blood-vessel constriction. This poor circulation and impaired nerve function increases the likelihood of numbness in the feet; cold weather further increases that likelihood, which can lead to foot injury during exercise. Neurological problems may also impair sense of thirst, making dehydration more likely; such problems may also inhibit sweating and so increase the risk of heat stroke.

High impact exercise can break blood vessels in diseased eyes or injure a foot that is permanently numb due to nerve damage. Straining and holding the breath can break blood vessels in the diseased eye also.

- Client should take an exercise stress test before starting the exercise program, to rule out coronary disease.

- Keep heart rate below 70% of its maximum rate (220 – client's age).

- To prevent excessive absorption of injected insulin, client should inject it into muscle that won't be exercised, then wait at least 1 hour before exercising.

- Wait at least 1 hour after meals before exercising.

- Client should check blood sugar levels before and after workout; if necessary, adjust diet or insulin dosage to prevent excessive drop in sugar.

Carry sugar packets during workout, in case symptoms of low blood sugar are experienced.

### Guidelines for Type 1 Diabetics

The following steps are crucial for Type 1 diabetics to avoid hyperglycaemia or hypoglycaemia during and after exercise.

1. Ingest 40-60 grams of carbohydrate prior to exercise lasting up to 30 minutes. For exercise beyond 30 minutes, consume 15-30 grams carbohydrate for every 30 minutes of moderately intense exercise. A meal 1-3 hours before exercise is recommended.

2. Consume a snack of slowly absorbed carbohydrate (e.g. legumes, fructose, pasta, milk) following prolonged exercise sessions.

3. Reduce the insulin dose before exercise:

   a. *Intermediate-acting insulin.* Reduce by 30-35% on the day of exercise. Inject insulin at least 1 hour before exercise.

   b. *Short-acting insulin.* Omit dose of short-acting insulin that precedes exercise.

   c. *Continuous subcutaneous infusion.* Reduce mealtime increment when exercising just before or after a meal.

4. Avoid exercising the muscle area underlying injections of short-acting insulin for at least 1 hour.

5. Monitor blood glucose before, during, and after exercise.

6. Learn individual glucose responses to different types of exercise.

*Source:* Young JC. Exercise prescription for individuals with metabolic disorders: Practical considerations. *Sports Med* 19:43-53, 1995

## Benefits and Risks of Exercise for Individuals with Diabetes

Diabetics must be cautious about the possible risk of exercise, but the possible benefits are great, as well.

### Possible Benefits

1. Decreased food glucose

2. Increased insulin sensitivity

3. Improved blood lipoprotein profile and lowered blood pressure

4. Improved cardiorespiratory fitness

5. Usefulness as adjunct to diet for weight reduction

6. Increased sense of well-being and quality of life.

### Possible Risks

1. Hypoglycaemia during or after exercise

2. Increased blood glucose values among poorly controlled patients.

3. Complications of atherosclerotic cardiovascular disease

4. Degenerative joint disease

5. Worsening of diabetic complications.

*Source:* Young JC. Exercise prescription for individuals with metabolic disorders: Practical considerations. *Sports Med* 19:43-53, 1995.

### Arthritis

Warming up loosens stiff muscles and joints. After each workout it is important to stretch in order to maintain joint mobility by keeping muscles from contracting. Cold weather can stiffen joints and muscles and high-impact exercise can damage arthritic joints. A safety measure would be to avoid pushing past the range of motion and injuring joints.

- Client should only stretch and not exercise when pain or inflammation is worse than usual.

- Try aerobic exercise only if client can do easier exercises, such as stretching or light strength training, without pain.

- Choose maximum intensity that causes no significant discomfort, including pain during workout and aches that persist for more than about 24 hours after workout.

- Client should consider doing calisthenics (in a heated pool) or T'ai Chi, which can safely stretch and strengthen all major joints.

**Osteoporosis**

There are no special warm ups or cool downs for osteoporosis but exercising in any chilly or icy conditions can cause bone-breaking falls. Whereas high impact exercise is of general importance to stimulate bone growth in osteoporosis, there is also the danger of cracking thin bones. This is also the case for using free weights if strength or balance is poor.

- Vertebrae of the back can be stressed and fractured so any manoeuvres which over-work this area need to be avoided.

- Avoid significant discomfort through maximum intensity in a workout which might also cause pain which persists for more than 24 hours after exercise.

- If there is a risk of falling during an exercise program, then it should be avoided.

- Bicycling and swimming should be exchanged for more weight-bearing exercise which will put a little more pressure on the hips and spine.

## Asthma

The likelihood of an asthma attack is reduced by warming up which allows warm air to enter the lungs. In cooling down it is important not to stop abruptly so that an asthma attack is triggered. Cold air or polluted air, especially when dry, can trigger or worsen an attack. There are no special warnings or considerations in regard to high-impact exercise.

- The client should drink water before, during, and after workout, even in cool weather, to moisten airways.

- If exercise triggers asthma attacks, medication should be taken before a workout and carried during the workout.

- Exercise should not be close to busy roads.

- The client should cover the mouth with a mask or scarf when exercising in cold, to heat and humidify air.

- For aerobic exercise, the client may consider swimming because high humidity near water helps prevent attacks.

## Lifestyle Factors That Reduce Low-Density Lipoprotein Cholesterol (LDL-C) and Total Cholesterol

It has been shown that people who exercised for 3 x 10-minute sessions a day present greater improvements in blood cholesterol levels than those who exercise for half an hour in a single session.

The following factors are listed in approximate order of importance.

1. Reduction of dietary saturated fat intake (especially meat and dairy fats) and of intake of trans fatty acids (mainly from hydrogenated fats)

2. Reduction in body weight

3. Reduction in dietary cholesterol intake (found in all animal foods)

4. Increase in dietary polyunsaturated and mono-unsaturated fatty acids (mainly from plant foods, fish, and olives)

5. Increase in carbohydrate and dietary water-soluble fibres (especially fruits and vegetables, beans, and oat products)

6. Control of stress (weak evidence)

7. Reduction of dietary caffeine, coffee consumption (weak evidence)

## Physical Activity Alleviates Obesity

To sustain successful body fat loss, it is necessary to burn about 4,000 calories a week which is equivalent to walking 65km/40 miles a week and regular exercise is the key to maintaining healthy body fat levels. Accumulating physical activity is considered more successful for obese clients than providing a structured exercise program.

## CHAPTER SIXTEEN: Exercise and cognitive impairment:

Exercise has extraordinary benefits for older adults including those with disabilities and assists in reducing the risk of developing secondary conditions that arise from physical disuse and functional decline. With age, the incidence of dementia increases and this also impacts on people's ability to maintain occupational and social functioning. Alzheimer's disease is the most prevalent and devastating form of dementia and dementia sufferers can live up to 20 years as it advances.

Regular exercise that focuses on function fitness, such as walking, has been associated with significant reductions in the levels of dependence and disability in older adults. The relationship between physical fitness levels, specifically aerobic fitness, cognition, and physical health in older adults, is well established. There is also empirical support for exercise improving physical fitness, behaviour, cognition, communication, and functioning in older people with cognitive impairments.

Various studies have revealed that exercise can be effective when used with rehabilitation programs for cognitive impairment, dementia, Alzheimer's disease and geriatric fields. Fitness, physical function, cognitive function and positive behaviour are increased in this special population when carried out on a systematic basis.

Aerobic fitness training comes out strongly as a form of exercise which helps to reduce brain tissue loss as people get older. This also has a positive effect on cognitive function and lowers the risk of developing Alzheimer's disease and other related cognitive disorders compared with a sedentary population of ageing people.

The association of the development of Alzheimer's disease and related disorders with similar risk factors for heart disease and stroke – points to conditions such as hyperlipidaemia. It has also been found that in countries where there is a high dietary fat consumption, there is also a high level of dementia. The assumption then is that designing physical exercises to prevent and manage cardiovascular disease and hypertension should also be very effective in preventing dementia.

The most unfortunate aspect of cognitive decline and disorders is that people often require long-term care which is usually offered in a nursing home environment. Institutionalised settings rarely provide the opportunity for physical activities and the environment may also lack mental and cognitive stimulation, hastening a decline in the aged person.

**Physical Exercise and Psychological Health.**

There are many potential psychological benefits for people suffering from psychiatric disorders as well as the aged and unfit, when they commence low intensity exercise programs. In several studies it has been shown that low or moderate-intensity activities bring about a sound improvement to mental health. It has also been shown that aerobic exercise combined with counselling is considerably more effective than counselling alone for treatment of depressive disorders. Depression is compounded in physically inactive people compared to individuals who exercise regularly.

**Exercise Alleviates Depression**

Mood-enhancing benefits come from regular, moderate exercise especially when it is done outdoors. Research has shown that a 20 minute walk on the beach or through woodland can reduce stress. The brainwave frequency can also be altered to stress-reducing alpha waves and is often more effective than medication and psychotherapy in fighting depression.

## CHAPTER SEVENTEEN:   Exercise, immunity and aging.

There is always an added risk of infection in older age when protective aspects of the immune system cease to be effective.  Some recent studies of healthy centenarians who are examples of successful ageing have shown however, that there is a complex reshaping and remodelling of the immune system with age.  It was discovered through these studies that a regimen of endurance exercise which was appropriate might be used to assist the elderly in achieving an improved quality of life through enhancing the immune system.  During both rest and exercise the immune system is effected and influenced by many age-related changes which take place in the physiological systems.  Depending upon the type of exercise, there may be a multifaceted response from the immune system and significant interaction between the neuroendocrine and immune systems.  In theory, moderate exercise may help to reverse the adverse effect of ageing upon the immune system by increasing the production of endocrine hormones.  There would be less accumulation of autoreactive immune cells by enhancing the programmed cell death.  Again endurance training in later life increases resistance to both viral infections and the formation of malignant cells.  In order to avoid any adverse effects of exercise in an elderly population, it is important to evaluate and adjust any exercise program.  Exercise in mature years is also associated with the way in which circulating T cell functions and the related production of cytokine – so that age-related decline is reduced.

### Exercise Reverses Aging in Muscle

It is often a surprise to elderly people that they develop real enhanced muscle tissue when they commence an exercise program. They are able to carry out many tasks that had become difficult and also to reduce the risk of disability due to arthritis especially through resistance training which builds muscle tissue in a healthy  aged population.

With a decline in mitochondrial function in the aged, comes a loss of muscle mass as the powerhouse of the cell becomes dysfunctional.

Exercise has been shown to reverse the genetic profile to acquire similar levels of mitochondrial functioning to that seen in young adults  and research has shown that mitochondrial dysfunction was the most common 'theme'  to emerge from the gene expression profile.

The fact that the 'genetic fingerprints' so dramatically reversed course, gives credence to the value of exercise, not only as a means of improving health, but of reversing the aging process itself, which is an additional incentive to exercise as you get older. As well as creating a reversal of the muscle cell biology, healthy weight can be achieved and the reduction of risk for disabilities like arthritis. Further research hopes to establish whether endurance training such as walking or cycling can also impact in the same way on mitochondrial function and a reversal of the ageing process.

## Exercise, Mobility and Aging

As the 'baby boomers' moved on to older age, the growth of the elderly population also takes up a larger proportion of the total population. When elderly people experience poor health and immobility, this will also increase in the cost to the community. Independence and mobility for the elderly are understated goals which need to be taken up by the ageing population, trainers, medical practitioners, allied health consultants and politicians.

As well, impaired gait and balance pose significant risk factors for falls and mobility in the elderly. Exercise brings great benefits for various psychological and physiological parameters in an ageing populations and should be also a major focus for all in the aged care sector.

## Using exercise as the fountain of youth

Aging is inevitable, but there's no reason why the process can't be more enjoyable. Exercise can promise better health, functional independence and a better quality of life as you age, in fact it can help slow the aging process by preventing or reducing the chances of disease and disability as seniors.

The body is a time machine, beautifully crafted, exquisitely functional and temperamental, responding to every internal and external stimulus. The level of respect and the knowledge and care of this machine will go far to increase its longevity and workings. Each cell has its own intelligence and cells are martialled to work together or against certain stimuli.

The body as an art form is celebrated for its beauty and aesthetic qualities. This is so elementary and necessary to attract attention to it and to at least love it for external appearances. Aesthetics can and should stimulate health without excessively dominating the reasons for having a beautiful form – for essentially beauty comes from within.

The true artistry of the body, lies in its superb performance, as Leonardo da Vinci discovered in the most painstaking way. Although generations of scholarly physiologists have revealed the workings of the body to us, we carry around this wonderful machine without knowing how to fully operate it, let alone maintain it. We accept age and infirmity before taking further responsibility. Yet the body and its complex multiple functioning accept challenges so readily. Do we understand how the nervous system warns or prepares us for activity? How blood is shunted from one receptive site to another within the body? The communication between cells and the collapse of the immune system when stress takes over? The real meaning of 'shock' when the body shuts down and ceases to function resulting in death. How can we grow strong bones again at an older age or gain defined and strong muscles? Years do not have to equal lack of mobility, strength and energy.

Exercising over 50 can give the individual fitness, health, peace of mind and joy. The confidence gained will also go a long way to experiencing long term mobility and independence.

# Counteracting Iatrogenic Disease With Targeted Exercise Prescriptions

| Disease(s) | Standard Treatment | Unintended Side Effect | Exercise Recommendation |
|---|---|---|---|
| Acute or chronic pain syndromes | Narcotic analgesics | Constipation | Aerobic training Progressive resistance training |
| Chronic renal failure | Low-protein diet | Decreased lean body mass | Progressive resistance training |
| Chronic liver disease | | Decreased albumin, Diminished growth hormone, IGF-1, Muscle weakness | Progressive resistance training |
| Congestive heart failure | Digoxin | Anorexia | Progressive Resistance training |
| Atrial fibrillation | | | Aerobic training |
| Coronary artery disease | Alpha- and beta-blockers, calcium channel blockers, anticholinergics, antidepressant, diuretics, other cardiac medications. | Orthostatic hypotension, falls, hip fractures | Progressive resistance training |
| Hypertension | Antihypertensives (alpha-blockers, beta-blockers, reserpine) | Depression | Aerobic training, progressive resistance training |
| Parkinson's disease | | | Balance training |
| Oedema | Diuretics | Urinary incontinence | Kegel pelvic floor isometric strengthening exercises. |

| | | | |
|---|---|---|---|
| Depression | Antidepressants (tricyclics, selective serotonin reuptake inhibitors) | Postural hypotension, falls, hip fractures | Balance training, Progressive resistance training. |
| Epilepsy | Anticonvulsants | Osteomalacia | Progressive resistance training |
| Osteoporosis | | | Weight-bearing aerobic training, high-velocity, high-impact loading (e.g. jumping) |
| Fracture of appendicular bone | Casting, immobilization in splint | Muscle atrophy | Isometric contractions under cast while immobilized, progressive resistance training after removal of cast |
| Hypothyroidism | Thyroxine | Osteoporosis | Progressive resistance training, weight-bearing aerobic training, high-velocity, high-impact loading, e.g. jumping. |
| Insomnia | Benzodiazepines | Impaired motor coordination, gait, and balance | Balance training |
| Major surgery | Operative procedure. Bed rest | Catabolism, Muscle wasting | Progressive resistance training |
| Rheumatic diseases | Corticosteroids | Proximal myopathy | Progressive resistance training |
| Immunosupression for organ transplant. | | Osteoporosis, visceral fat deposition | Progressive resistance training |
| Chronic obstructive | | Insulin resistance, hyperglycaemia, | Progressive resistance |

| pulmonary disease | | increased blood pressure, hypertension | training. |
|---|---|---|---|
| Obesity | Energy restriction | Decreased lean body mass (muscle and bone) | Progressive resistance training. |

Fiatarone Singh, M.A., 2002, 'Exercise Comes of Age: 'Rationale and Recommendations for a Geriatric Exercise Prescription', *Journal of Gerontology: MEDICAL SCIENCES,* Vol 57A, No. 5, M262-M282.

# BIBLIOGRAPHY

Egger, G., Champion, N., & Bolton, A., 1998, *The Fitness Leader's Handbook,* Kangaroo Press, Kenthurst, NSW.

Hall, J. 2002, *The Exercise Bible,* Kyle Cathie Ltd. UK.

Shephard, R.J., 1997, *Aging, physical activity and health.* Human Kinetics, Champaign.

St. George, F., 2002, *Bodyworks,* Francine St George, The Physiotherapy, Posture and Fitness Clinic, Sydney

# ARTICLES

Babyak, M., Blumenthal, J.A., Herman, St., Khatri, P., Doraiswamy, M., Moore, K., Edward Craighead, W., Baldewicz., T.T., Ranga Krishnan, K., 2000, 'Exercise Treatment for Major Depression: Maintenance of Therapeutic Benefit at 10 Months', *Psychosom Med,* Vol. 62 No. 5, September/October.

Blumenthal, J.A., Babyak, M.A., Moore, K.A., Craighead, W.E., Herman, S., Khatri, P., Waugh, R., Napolitano, M.A., Forman, L.M., Appelbaum, M., Doraiswamy, P.M., Krishnan, K.R., 1999, 'Effects of exercise training on older patients with major depression', *Internal Medicine,* Vol. 159, No. 19, 25 October.

Daley, M.J., Spinks, W.L., 2000, 'Exercise, mobility and aging', *Sports Med* Jan Vol. 29. No. 1 pp 1-12.

Evans, W.J., Cyr-Campbell, D., 1997, 'Nutrition, exercise, and healthy aging', *Journal of the American Dietetic Association*, pp. 632-638.

'Exercise and aging: Can you walk away from Father Time? (This article was first printed in the December 2005 issue of the Harvard Men's Health Watch) *http://www.health.harvard.edu/newsletters/Harvard_Mens_Health_Watch.htm*.)

Fiatarone Singh, M.A., 2002, 'Exercise Comes of Age: Rationale and Recommendations for a Geriatric Exercise Prescription', *Journal of Gerontology: MEDICAL SCIENCES,* Vol. 57A, No. 5, M262-M282.

Gluckman, G., 1995, 'Muscle Balance and Function Development', *B.C. Massage Practitioner*, Fall.

Greist, J.H., Klein, M.H., Eischens, R.R., Faris, J., Gurman, A.S. & Morgan W.P., 1979, 'Running as Treatment for Depression', *Comprehensive Psychiatry,* Vol. 20, No. 1, January-February.

Heyn, P., Abreu, B.C., Ottenbacher, K.J., 2004, 'The Effects of Exercise Training on Elderly Persons With Cognitive Impairment and Dementia: A Meta-Analysis', *Arch Phys Med Rehabil,* Vol. 85, October.

Hurley, B.F., Roth, S.M., 2000, 'Strength Training in the Elderly: Effects on Risk Factors for Age-Related Diseases', *Sports Medicine,* Vol. 30, No. 4, October, pp 249-268.

Klein, M.H., Greist, J.H., Gurman, A.S., Neimeyer, R.A., Lesser, D.P., Bushnell, N.J., Smith, R.E., 1985, 'A Comparative Outcome Study of Group Psychotherapy vs Exercise Treatments for Depression', *Int. J. Ment. Health.,* Vol. 13, No 3-4, pp. 148-177.

Mather, A.S., Rodriguez, C., Guthrie, M.F., McHarg, A.M., Reid, I.C., McMurdo, M.E.T., 2002, 'Effects of exercise on depressive symptoms in older adults with poorly responsive depressive disorder', *British Journal of Psychiatry,* Vol. 180 pp 411-415.

Martinsen, E.W., Hoffaret, A., Solberg, O., 1989, 'Comparing aerobic with nonaerobic forms of exercise in the treatment of clinical depression: A randomized trial', *Comprehensive Psychiatry,* Vol. 30, No. 4 (July/August), pp 324-331.

McNeil, J.K., LeBlanc, E.M., Joyner, M., 1991, 'The effect of exercise on depressive symptoms in the moderately depressed elderly', *Psychology and Aging,* Vol 6, No. 3, pp. 487-488.

Melov, S., Tarnopolsky, M., McMaster University Medical Center in Hamilton, Ontario, led a team to analyse gene expression involved in age-related mitochondrial function.

Nied, R.J., Franklin, B., 2002, 'Promoting and prescribing exercise for the elderly, *Am Fam Physician,* 1:65(3) pp 419-427

Shephard, R.J., 1998, 'Aging and Exercise', In: Encyclopedia of Sports Medicine and Science, T.D. Fahey (Editor). *Internet Society for Sport Science: http://sportsci.org.* 7 March.

Singh, N.A., Clements, K.M., Fiatarone Singh, M.A., 2001, 'The Efficacy of Exercise as a Long-term Antidepressant in Elderly Subjects: A Randomized, Controlled Trial', *Journal of Gerontology: MEDICAL SCIENCES,* Vol. 56A, No. 8 M497-M504.

'The Discovery of Endorphins', 2002, *http://www.methadone.org/discover.html*

Veale, D., Le Fevre, K., Pantelis, C., de Souza, V., Mann, A., Sargeant, A., 1992, 'Aerobic exercise in the adjunctive treatment of depression: a randomized controlled trial', *Journal of the Royal Society of Medicine,* Vol. 85, September.

Venjatraman J.T., Fernandes, G., 1997. 'Exercise, immunity and aging', *Aging (Milan, Italy6),* 9(1-2) 42-56

Waehner, P., 2011, 'Aging and Exercise – Combat the Effects of Aging with Exercise – Using exercise as your fountain of youth', *About.com Guide,* March 15.

Weyerer, S., Kupfer, B. 1994, 'Physical Exercise and Psychological Health', *Sports Medicine,* Feb. Vol 17. No. 2 pp 108-116/

Willett, S., 2002, 'Runner's High', http:///lehigh.edu/~dmd1/sarah.html

Young, J.C.,1995, 'Exercise prescription for individuals with metabolic disorders: Practical considerations', *Sports Med* 19:43-53.

## PERSONAL INTERVIEWS

Ann Cusack, Personal Trainer, Sydney 2013

John 'Sparrow' Dowse, Fitness Trainer, Sydney, 2013

Diane Gosden, Tai Chi Teacher and Practitioner, Sydney 2013

David Gosden, Ocean Swimmer, Sydney 2013

## SPINAL FLEXIBILITY & STRETCHING EXERCISES CHART

Source: Dr. Kevin Unterreriner

# SPINAL FLEXIBILITY & STRETCHING EXERCISES

Helps to build strong muscles to support your neck and back. STRETCHING EXERCISES increase flexibility and movement of the joints of the body and spine. Do exercises 5 to 10 times, 3 times a week, and don't do any that cause pain.

## LYING

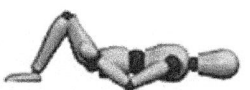

Bend knees, lie on back, take a deep breath, place your hands on your thighs and relax.

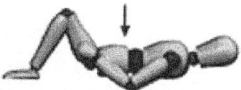

Tighten your abdomen and buttocks. Press your lower back onto the floor. ACTION — Stretches and strengthens stomach and back muscles.

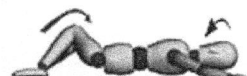

Turn both knees to one side while rotating your head to the opposite side. ACTION — stretches lower back, mid back, muscles, and joints.

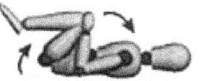

Pull both knees to your chest. ACTION — stretches lower back, buttocks and abdominal muscles.

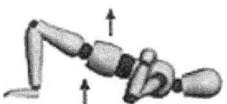

Slowly raise hips upward. Keep a straight line from the knees to the shoulders. Do not arch your back. ACTION — stretches buttocks and stretches upper leg muscles.

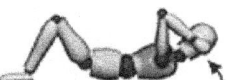

Cross your arms, tuck your chin in, tighten abdomen, and curl halfway up. Use hands behind head for support only. (Do not pull). ACTION — strengthens abdominal muscles.

## LYING

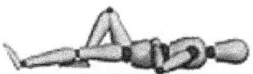

Lie on your back with one leg bent and the foot flat on the floor. Extend the opposite leg straight out. Relax and allow your back to feel the floor.

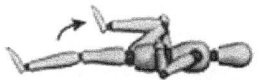

With knee bent, pull it to your chest, keeping the opposite leg straight, press your knee and lower back to the floor. ACTION — buttocks muscles, back muscles and stretches hip.

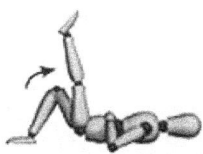

Press your lower back against the floor, raise the straight leg until it is level with the bent knee. ACTION — strengthens and stretches quadricep muscles, hamstring muscles and stretches hip joints.

## PRONE

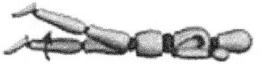

Lie on your stomach, raise one leg off the floor, while keeping the knee straight. ACTION — strengthens lower back, abdominal and leg muscles, stretches hamstrings and quadriceps.

Keep your neck in a normal position, push yourself up on your forearms. Keep hips and abdomen against floor. ACTION — strengthens posterior back muscles, attains normal low back curve.

## HANDS & KNEES

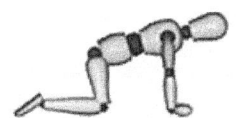

While on your hands and knees, keep your knees directly under your hips, your hands under your shoulders, keep abdominal muscles firm, keep your neck relaxed and in its normal position, that is, with your ears in line with your shoulders.

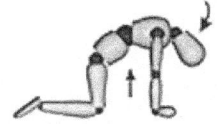

Drop your head down and press your back upwards by tightening your abdominal and buttocks muscles. ACTION — to strengthen abdominal and buttocks muscles and to stretch your lower and mid back.

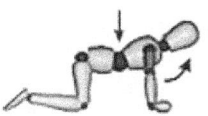

Relax your stomach and buttocks muscles and allow your back to sag. Do not sit back on your hips. ACTION — to stretch back and abdominal muscles and help maintain lower back curve.

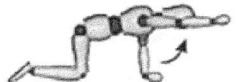

Stretch one arm straight out in front of you while maintaining your back and head position while keeping support arm straight. ACTION — strengthens and stretches your shoulder, upper back muscles and joints.

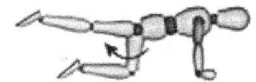

Extend your straight leg behind you while holding it parallel to the floor. Maintain your normal back and neck position. ACTION — strengthens buttocks, abdomen and leg muscles.

## NECK FLEX

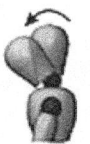

Drop head forward, slowly. You will feel the stretch of your neck muscles.

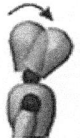

Slowly drop head backward and you will feel the stretch of your front neck muscles.

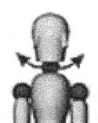

Slowly turn your head from side to side. Feel the stretch of the muscles on the side of your neck. Do not strain.

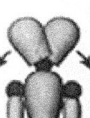

Tilt your head to one side. This is to stretch the muscles on the side of your neck.

## NECK STRENGTH

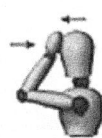

Press forehead to palm. Resist forward motion.

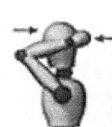

Clasp hands behind head, press your head back. resist motion.

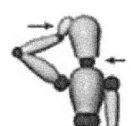

Turn head to one side, resist side motion with your hand.

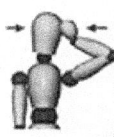

Tilt head to other side, resist motion with hand.

Name:                      D O B:

Address:               Postcode:

Email:                     Mobile:

## Physical Activity Readiness Questionnaire (PAR-Q)

If you are between the ages of 15 and 69, the PAR-Q will tell you if you should check with your doctor before you significantly change your physical activity patterns. If you are over 69 years of age and are not used to being very active, check with your doctor. Common sense is your best guide when answering these questions. Please read carefully and answer each one honestly: check YES or NO.

| | | Yes | No |
|---|---|---|---|
| 1. | Has your doctor ever said you have a heart condition and that you should only do physical activity recommended by a doctor? | ☐ | ☐ |
| 2. | Do you feel pain in your chest when you do physical activity? | ☐ | ☐ |
| 3. | In the past month, have you had a chest pain when you were not doing physical activity? | ☐ | ☐ |
| 4. | Do you lose you balance because of dizziness or do you ever lose conciousness? | ☐ | ☐ |
| 5. | Do you have a bone or joint problem (for example, back, knee, or hip) that could be made worse by a change in your physical activity? | ☐ | ☐ |
| 6. | Is your doctor currently prescribing medication for your blood pressure or heart condition? | ☐ | ☐ |
| 7. | Do you know of any other reason why you should not do physical activity? | ☐ | ☐ |

If yes, please comment: _____

**YES to one or more questions:**
You should consult with your doctor to clarify that it is safe for you to become physically active at this current time and in your current state of health.

**NO to all questions:**
It is reasonably safe for you to participate in physical activity, gradually building up from your current ability level. A fitness appraisal can help determine your ability levels.

**I have read, understood and accurately completed this questionnaire. I confirm that I am voluntarily engaging in an acceptable level of exercise, and my participation involves a risk of injury.**

Signature _____

Print name _____

Date _____

**Having answered YES to one of the above, I have sought medical advice and my GP has agreed that I may exercise.**

Signature _____

Date _____

**Note:** This physical activity clearance is valid for a maximum of 12 months from the date it is completed and becomes invalid if your condition changes so that you would answer YES to any of the 7 questions.

# Exercise Log

Date:

Time:

Location:

Instructor:

Type of Workout:

Duration/Intensity:

Focus:

How I Felt Before:

How I Felt After:

My Workout Notes:

My Future Goals:

# New Food Pyramid

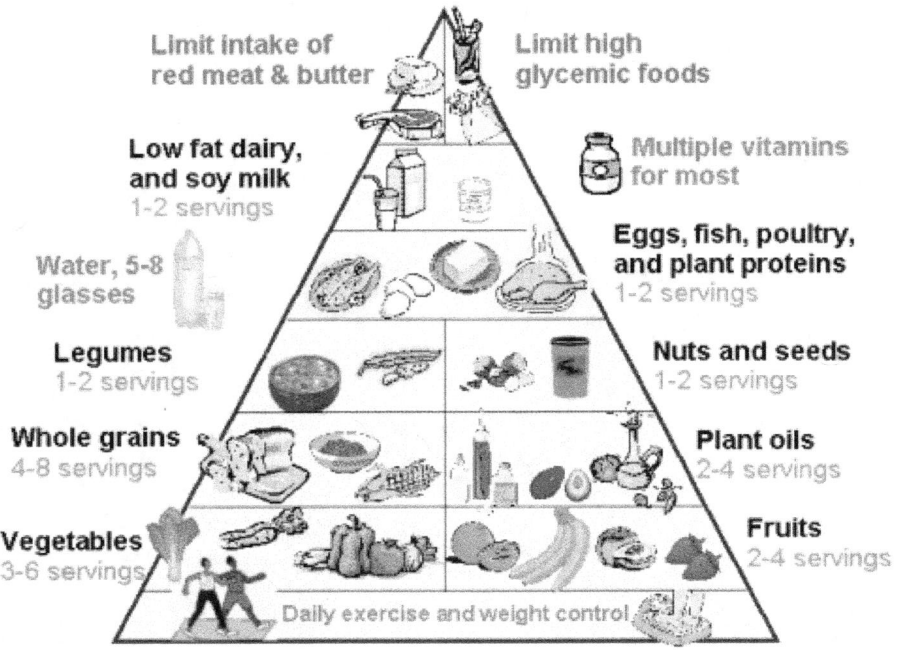

Limit intake of red meat & butter

Limit high glycemic foods

**Low fat dairy, and soy milk**
1-2 servings

Multiple vitamins for most

Water, 5-8 glasses

**Eggs, fish, poultry, and plant proteins**
1-2 servings

**Legumes**
1-2 servings

**Nuts and seeds**
1-2 servings

**Whole grains**
4-8 servings

**Plant oils**
2-4 servings

**Vegetables**
3-6 servings

**Fruits**
2-4 servings

Daily exercise and weight control

# EXERCISE PRESCRIPTION FOR CLIENT WITH OBESITY

**Health Screening Tools:**

- Pre-screening questionnaire (PAR-Q)
- Anthropometry – BMI, WHR and girth measurements
- Blood Pressure
- Resting heart rate
- VO2 max test

**Recommended precautions before, during and after exercise:**

**Before**

- Pre-screening (depending on results, check up with GP)
- Fitness assessment
- Warm up and stretching

**During**

- Check heart rate regularly
- Drink plenty of fluids
- No jarring exercises
- Monitor exercise regularly
- Monitor intensity

**After**

- Cool down and stretching
- Drink fluids
- Monitor heart rate
- Motivation and feed back

**Appropriate Exercises**

- Bike
- Rowing machine
- X-trainer
- Stepper
- Swimming
- Aqua aerobics
- Walking i.e. around a park or beach

**Resistance Training**

- Pin loaded machine (where appropriate)

- Some free weights

## Aerobic Exercise Protocol

- Frequency     2-4 sessions per week
- Duration     Initially 10-30 mins, review after 4-6 weeks
- Intensity     60-70% max heart rate, review 4-6 weeks, increase  capacity

## Weight Training Protocol

- Frequency     2-3 sessions per week
- Sets     1-2
- Reps     10-15
- Intensity     50% IRM
- Training     20-30 mins
- Recovery     Aerobic workout – recovery will occur between set exercises

## Motivational Strategies

- Food Diary
- Goal Setting with reassessment after 4-6 weeks
- Variety in Training Program

# EXERCISE PRESCRIPTION FOR CLIENT WITH DIABETES

**Precautions before Exercise**

- Test for fitness, retinopathy, circulation, nerve problems, PAR-Q test
- Check glucose levels before exercising and make sure client has sufficient carbohydrate storage
- Feet should be checked for blisters, cuts, Athlete's Foot
- Client should not inject muscle which is to be trained
- Exercise only 1-2 hours after eating.

**During Exercise**

- ID tag to be worn
- Closely monitor glucose levels, client should keep sugar packets, jelly beans
- Watch out for signs of glycaemia, increase in heart rate, fatigue or dizziness
- Keep well hydrated
- Avoid extreme weather conditions such as cold/wet weather which can lead to feet problems.

**Post Exercise**

- Check glucose levels and insulin
- Replenish glycogen stores
- Replace fluid loss
- Check feet for blisters, cuts etc.
- Client should monitor for delayed onset hypoglycaemia

**Types of Exercise**

- Aerobic exercise with progressive increase needed
- Keep to minimum impact exercises like cycling
- Resistance training – low weight, high reps
- In younger people, a more strenuous weight program can be adopted
- Intensity will vary according to past training experiences and fitness levels
- If blood vessels in the feet and eyes are damaged, avoid high impact cardio and strenuous weights
- Life style changes e.g. taking the stairs instead of the lift

**Aerobic Exercise Protocol**

- Frequency: 4-7 times per week
- Duration: minimum 20 minutes but try to increase to 60 mins.

- Intensity:  Type 1 Diabetes should seek medical clearance before commencing a program
- Assuming health is average, work at 75% of max heart rate or 70% VO2Max
- Also can use RPE (rate of perceived exertion) such as the BORG scale 6-20 and work on client feedback
- Gentle warm up and cool down
- Stretching, especially muscles that need to be exercised
- Not too hard an impact  on the feet like running on hard surfaces
- Avoid high impact classes such as Step classes

## Motivational Strategies

- Give positive feedback after sessions with client
- Refer back to original fitness testing and look for improvements in client fitness and loss of body fat
- Always encourage clients to do their best but not to overwork themselves
- Also consider goal setting such as a small event or to better their times in training or increased resistance training workload
- Keep it fun and focussed
- Encourage lifestyle change with diet and incidental exercise  such as taking the stairs instead of a lift and walking instead of driving where possible
- Courtesy calls to clients after sessions to get feedback.

# EXERCISE PRESCRIPTION FOR CLIENT WITH OSTEOPOROSIS

## Health Screening Tools

- PAR-Q – or similar screening test
- One-minute Osteoporosis risk test

## Recommended Precautions Before/During/After Exercise

- Ensure that the muscles are warm and well stretched
- During exercise – steps must be taken to ensure that the client is not at risk of falling or becoming unbalanced increasing the risk of further injury i.e. floor coverings and equipment must be in working order
- During exercise the weight provided should not be too heavy or isolated to the one area or joint
- During exercise twisting of the spine and bending at the waist exercise should be avoided
- After exercise client must ensure that they cool down to prevent aching in the joints or bones

## Types of Exercise Considered Appropriate

- **Weight-bearing exercises**
- Walking
- Stationary exercise cycle
- Swimming (non-weight bearing)
- **Resistance Training**
- Resistance machines
- Free weights
- Body weights resistance

## Aerobic Exercise Protocol

- Frequency          4-7 times per week
- Intensity          The exercise should be at the highest level
- Duration          20-60 minutes depending on client fitness

## Weight Training Protocol

- Frequency          2-3 times per week in conjunction with aerobics
- Sets          2-3 sets
- Repetition range          10-15 reps
- Intensity          Power training – high intensity

- Training volume     5 exercises per training session
- Recovery time     60-90 secs between sets

## Motivational Strategies

- Fulfil  client's personal needs/goals
- Set milestones to be achieved
- Advancement – measurement of success
- Maintain or improve client's health and well being
- Responding to the client's fear of their medical condition.

# EXERCISE PRESCRIPTION FOR CLIENT WITH HYPERTENSION

## Screening Tools

- Sphygmanometer
- Stethoscope
- Letter of clearance from a general practitioner
- Pre-exercise questionnaire
- Fitness assessment – BMI, weight, girth measurements.

## Precautions Before, During and After Exercise

- Client should do 10 minutes of warm up at a light walking pace
- Client must never hold breath – this raises blood pressure
- When doing resistance training, client must be lifting light weight, not going on to failure
- Client must cool down – helps prevent sudden dangerous drop in blood pressure
- Client should consume plenty of water – fluid loss from heavy sweating causes potentially dangerous drop in blood pressure and increases risk of possible blood clots
- No overhead presses
- No high impact or strenuous exercises which can place excessive demands on heart
- Heart rate must be kept below 60% of maximum heart rate

## Appropriate Exercises

- Light calisthenics
- Marching on the spot
- Light weights
- Walking
- Slow jogging
- Swimming
- Cycling

## Aerobics Exercise Protocol – Frequency, Duration and Intensity

- Frequency            2-3 times a week increasing slowly to 4-5
- Duration             start with 20 minute periods depending on history
- Intensity             let the client decide on his/her level of comfort/Borg scale

## Weight Training Protocol – Frequency, Duration and Intensity

- Frequency — 2-3 times per week
- Duration — start with 20 minute periods depending on history
- Sets — 2-3 sets
- Repetitions — 10 with light weight
- Intensity — must be set to client's individual condition
- Training Volume — 30 minutes
- Recovery Between Sets – up to 2 minutes with light stretching

**Motivational Strategies**

- Goal orientation towards cardiovascular improvement
- Setting achievable goals
- Regular assessments
- Monitoring blood pressure regularly
- Positive approach towards the client.

# EXERCISE PRESCRIPTION FOR CLIENT WITH DYSLIPIDEMIA

Dyslipidemia – abnormalities of blood fats (high cholesterol, triglycerides and low HDL cholesterol) are major risk factors for vascular disease of the heart, kidneys, eyes and legs.  Regular exercise reduces cholesterol and triglyceride levels and raises HDL cholesterol.

## Health Screening Tools

- Par-Q test
- Blood pressure
- Girth measurements
- Letter from General Practitioner to cover training and weights
- Blood tests

## Precautions Before, During and After Exercise

- Check blood pressure
- Use a variety of sub maximal aerobic tests to determine fitness levels
- Constantly monitor heart rate and intensity throughout session
- Avoid movements that may cause blood pressure to rise
- Allow suitable cool down exercise and monitor for any pain in chest or abnormalities.

## Appropriate Exercise Prescription

- Aerobic exercise :  walking, jogging,
- Moderate intensity,
- Resistance training, bike, boxercise depending on fitness levels
- 60% aerobic, 40% resistance training with the focus on compound exercises

## Aerobic Exercise Protocol

- Frequency        3-5 times a week
- Duration         35 minutes of aerobic training
- Intensity        Begin at a low intensity and work towards angina, cool

## Weight Training Protocol

- Frequency        3-5 times per week
- Duration         25 minutes approximately
- Intensity        Moderate
- Sets             2-3 sets of each exercise
- Repetitions      12-15 repetitions with a medium training volume
- Recovery time    1-2 minutes between sets depending upon client

## Motivational Strategies

- Set goals and physical objectives for client to work towards
- Take girth measurements, weight to show client progress
- Monitor fitness progress – both aerobic and resistance training
- Discuss relevant health issues for cholesterol with client
- Reward strategies for good results and reassure client.

# EXERCISE PRESCRIPTION FOR CLIENT WITH OSTEOARTHRITIS

## Health Screening Tools

**Questionnaire** – used to identify factors associated with the cause and potential onset of osteoarthritis.

### Key Factors:

- Age (with particular attention to over 45's)
- Obesity/overweight (a visual appraisal should determine this)
- Occupation (look for repetitive stress movements that may have worn out joints, such as manual work, typing etc.)
- Sporting and activity history (Rugby, tennis, skiing, high impact aerobics, road running etc.)
- Previous joint injuries (especially knee, elbow and shoulder problems)
- Level of current activity (This will help to determine how much strength the muscles have to support the joint)
- Gender (more women suffer from arthritis than men).

**Postural Analysis** – check for a slouch and poor spinal alignment which may cause unnatural wear and tear of the joints.

## Recommended Precautions Before/During and After Exercise

- Consult with a medical practitioner before beginning a strength training program
- Warm up before strength training to avoid exercising
- Cut back on strength training during periods of acute inflammation
- Evaluate pain the day after exercise, and make appropriate adjustments to avoid overtraining
- Avoid overemphasis on specific areas, and work toward comprehensive muscle conditioning
- Protect stressed joints by using machines or wrist straps, for example, rather than gripping barbells with arthritic fingers
- Organise the training program when appropriate to avoid unnecessary movements between exercise stations or to avoid sitting and standing exercises
- Use proper posture to enhance joint function during strength exercise (Tips derived from, W. Westcott (1999) 'Strength Training for Seniors' in *Human Kinetics,* USA.)
- Take warm baths before and after work-outs to soothe joints
- Women should limit wearing high-heeled shoes
- Some food experts suggest a diet which includes omega-3 fatty oils, olive oil, cod liver oil and garlic to relive the symptoms of osteoarthritis.

### Types of Appropriate Exercise

- There is no evidence that normal physical activity can cause arthritis. Aquarobics, hydrotherapy and swimming have been demonstrated to be a benefit to arthritis sufferers while inappropriate weight bearing or impact exercises may aggravate symptoms.
- Exercises that strengthen the thigh muscles tend to protect the knees
- Jogging moderate distances does not appear to increase the risk of knee osteoarthritis but avoid activities that place a lot of stress on the knee including kneeling and deep-seated squats.
- Tai-Chi is a useful form of exercise for people with arthritis because it builds strength, flexibility and balance without placing a lot of stress on the joints (*The Arthritis Foundation of Australia* promotes a video ' Tai Chi for Arthritis' produced by Dr Paul Lam)

### Aerobic Exercise Protocol: Frequency, Duration and Intensity

Water based exercise is appropriate as a daily activity for those suffering from osteoarthritis. The buoyancy effect will ease the pain of gravity and body weight on the inflamed joint. The concentric nature of hydro-resistance will minimise the strain on muscles around joints but keep them conditioned and functioning. Duration of sessions should be no more than 45 mins for those with advanced conditions. The intensity can be varied but as long as pain is not too great, the client can work to his or her aerobic limit.

### Weight Training Protocol: Frequency, Sets, Repetition, Range, Intensity, Training Volume and Recovery Between Sets

A Tufts University study in 1994 found that a 12 week strength training eased the pain of osteoarthritis and rheumatoid arthritis. Program participants performed all of the strength exercises at 80% of their maximum resistance – a relatively high training intensity.

'Most strength exercises can be modified to decrease arthritic discomfort and increase ease of execution' Janie Clark, 1997 President, American Senior Fitness Association.

- Machine training may be preferred over free weights, since machines provide supportive structures and include fewer exercises that require firm gripping.
- If an exercise causes joint pain that persists for more than one hour it should be replaced.
- Brief exercise sessions are better tolerated than long work-outs
- Try shorter sessions of resistance or cardio on a different day rather than combining both in a longer session (e.g. 35 min sessions rather than 60 mins)
- Give muscle groups normal recovery period of at least 48 hours between sessions.

# EXERCISE PRESCRIPTION FOR CLIENT WITH DEPRESSION

## Screening Tools

The term depression is used to cover a broad range of symptoms from clinical depression (a psychiatric illness assessed by a psychiatrist for disability classification, medication and treatment) – to reactive depression and extreme sadness assessed by psychologists using testing and counselling interventions.

Devise your own questionnaire or interview as psychology testing is often restricted and base it on what is useful for you to know and their indicators. Clients will usually tell you if they have a diagnosed depression with medication. Questions about prescribed medication may lead to disclosure of depression, sleep patterns, concentration, eating patterns and external factors such as divorce or bereavement.

## Recommended Precautions Before/During/After Training

- Before – advice from psychiatrists or general practitioner or psychologists treating client in regard to behaviour and medication
- Factors effecting training might be tiredness, poor concentration and showing up for training session
- After training – information on sleep and dietary improvements and praise and encouragement from the trainer.

## Appropriate Activities

- Walking
- Cycling,
- Swimming
- Rowing
- Skipping
- Running
- Boxing
- Aerobic classes
- Circuit training
- Weight lifting
- Team sports

Prescribe exercise which is achievable but challenging.

## Aerobic Exercise Program

- 10 mins easy walk, 20 minute jog – heart rate at 70%, 10 min walk cool down
- 5-10 min dynamic stretching, 45 min body combat class, 10 min stretchingcool down.

- Warm up easy 5 min swim, 2 laps breast stroke, 2 laps free style, 2 laps back stroke and repeat again, cool down 5 min slow easy swim.
- Scenic walk with friends in the bush, mountains or beach – take a picnic!

**Weight Training at Beginner's level for Sedentary Clients**

- Machine weights 2-3 times per week
- 3 sets each exercise
- 15-25 repetitions to train the client for muscular endurance – less weight more reps
- Intensity 80% to failure
- Recovery – 60 secs – longer for more fragile client

**Motivational strategies**

- Setting goals – give client new direction and something to live for
- Accentuate positives – reward client, give them a feeling of self fulfilment
- Reinforce what is important to client – find out their own aspirations
- Communicate – give compliments and find out how client is feeling
- Acknowledgement and compassion will help to relieve symptoms of depression for client.